TETRAPLEGIA
AND PARAPLEGIA

TETRAPLEGIA AND PARAPLEGIA

A Guide for Physiotherapists

Ida Bromley MBE MCSP
District Superintendent Physiotherapist
Hampstead Health District
The Royal Free Hospital
London

Illustrated by
JANET PLESTED AIIP AMPA

THIRD EDITION

CHURCHILL LIVINGSTONE
EDINBURGH LONDON MELBOURNE AND NEW YORK 1985

CHURCHILL LIVINGSTONE
Medical Division of Longman Group Limited

Distributed in the United States of America by Churchill
Livingstone Inc., 1560 Broadway, New York, N.Y. 10036, and
by associated companies, branches and representatives
throughout the world.

First edition 1976
Second edition 1981
Third edition 1985

ISBN 0-443-03233-5

British Library Cataloguing in Publication Data
Bromley, Ida
    Tetraplegia and paraplegia: a guide for physiotherapists. – 3rd ed.
    1. Quadriplegia   2. Paraplegia   3. Physical therapy
    I. Title
    616.8'37062   RC406.Q33

Library of Congress Cataloging in Publication Data
Bromley, Ida
    Tetraplegia and paraplegia.
    Bibliography: p. 00
    Includes index.
    1. Quadriplegia – Patients – Rehabilitation.   2. Paraplegia – Patients – Rehabilitation.
    3. Physical therapy.   I. Title.   [DNLM: 1. Paraplegia–therapy.   2. Physical Therapy
    3. Quadriplegia–therapy.
    WL 346 B868t]
    RC406.Q33B76   1985   616.8'37062   85–7786

Printed in Great Britain at The Bath Press, Avon

Preface to the Third Edition

In the past few years there have been a number of developments in the management of patients with spinal cord injury. This Third Edition contains added material which reflects these changes and parts of the text have been re-arranged to facilitate the use of the book.

The chapter on the medical background and the section on respiratory care have been revised. A more comprehensive, though not exhaustive chapter on the treatment of patients with incomplete lesions, concentrates on the management of spasticity. Pressure and its problems are brought together in one chapter. The functional, and motor innervation charts, with additional charts on sensory innervation, now form appendices for easy reference. Some recent research is reported and the remainder of the text has been updated as necessary.

Among the many people who have helped me, I would like to give special thanks to Miss Ebba Bergström and Dr Hans Frankel from Stoke Mandeville Hospital, Aylesbury, and Dr Michael Morgan from the Brompton Hospital, London. I am indebted to Miss Susan Edwards of the Royal Free Hospital, London, a colleague for many years, for Chapter 14, which has enlarged the scope of this book. The unfailing assistance, tolerance and good humour of the staff of Churchill Livingstone have been much appreciated thoughout the preparation of this edition.

London, 1985   I.B.

Preface to the First Edition

This book has been written in response to many requests from post-graduate and student physiotherapists in Great Britain and overseas. The aim has been to produce a manual for use in the practical situation.

The layout of certain sections may appear repetitious to the casual reader. However, I hope that the arrangement of material will facilitate the use of the book for those who are involved in handling the patients and who believe, as I do, that efficient treatment depends upon detail.

The principles of treatment were initially laid down by Sir Ludwig Guttmann at the National Spinal Injuries Centre. Sir Ludwig's interest in and enthusiasm for physiotherapy is well known, and I am indebted to him for being a patient teacher over the years.

In writing this book I am indebted to many people:

To Miss Elvira Hobson FCSP for permission to use the text for her book *Physiotherapy in Paraplegia*, which was the pioneer on this subject.

To all those in my own and allied professions who have criticised sections of the manuscript and given me their valuable and constructive help.

To Miss Pat Davies MCSP (Superintendent Physiotherapist, Kings College Hospital, London) and Mrs Gay Harrison MCSP (Deputy Superintendent Physiotherapist, Stoke Mandeville Hospital) for their patience in going through the entire manuscript and giving me unstintingly their time, criticism, and advice.

To my colleagues at Stoke Mandeville for their encouragement and their tolerance in repeatedly trying out the instructions for the functional activities, and to Mrs Peperell for her patient typing and re-typing of the manuscript.

I am specially grateful to Miss Jan Plested for her interest in and enthusiasm for her work on the illustrations. If this little book fulfils its function, I feel it will be largely due to her excellent diagrams.

Lastly I wish to thank members of the staff of Churchill Livingstone for their unfailing help and advice.

July, 1975   I.B.

Contents

1
Introduction

THE PURPOSE OF THE BOOK

Approximately 700 people in Great Britain fracture their spines every year and as a result remain totally or partially paralysed for the rest of their lives. In addition to these there are victims of spinal cord injury or disease from many other causes. 40 years ago such people died from the resulting complications. Today a normal life expectancy can be anticipated providing the correct treatment is given and the complications thus avoided.

It is the purpose of this book to give some guidelines to physiotherapists faced with the problem of treating patients with tetraplegia or paraplegia. These patients, who are initially totally dependent on those around them, need expert care and training if they are to become independent once again. It is an exciting challenge to be involved in and contribute to the metamorphosis which occurs when a tetraplegic or paraplegic patient evolves into a spinal man (Fig. 1.1).

Maximum detail has been given in the sections dealing with the tetraplegic patient. Solutions to the majority of problems facing those with paraplegia have now been found, whereas the social, professional and industrial rehabilitation of those with tetraplegia still leaves much to be desired.

The tetraplegic patient needs a longer period of rehabilitation to achieve his maximum independence. He needs a team around him who will not give up easily, but who are willing to persevere to overcome the sometimes apparently insurmountable obstacles. The treatments given in the following chapters are suggestions only, some methods which have been tried and found successful in certain cases. They are in no way given as the total answer, but simply as a foundation on which other physiotherapists can build. They are initial guidelines only to encourage others to search for ways of achieving greater independence, whether physical or mechanical, for those with tetraplegia.

REHABILITATION

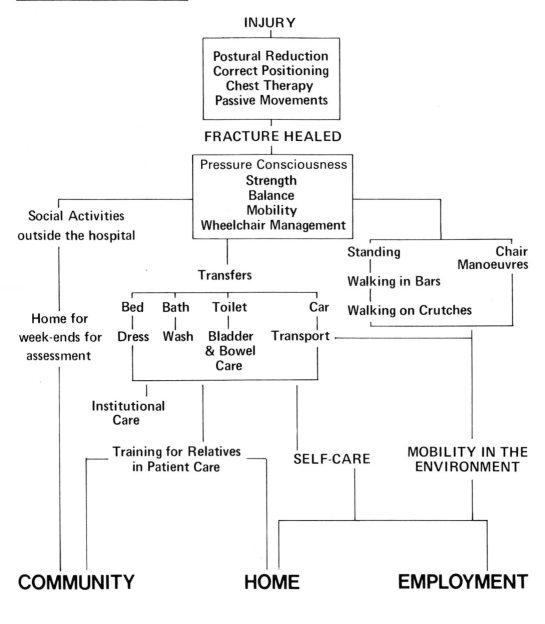

Fig. 1.1 Dependence to independence.

SPINAL CORD INJURIES

Of the cases admitted to spinal units approximately 70% are traumatic, and approximately 50% of these involve the cervical spine.

The majority of the traumatic cases, approximately 50%, are the result of road traffic accidents. Industrial accidents account for approximately 26%, sporting injuries 10%, and accidents in the home approximately 10%. The majority of the traumatic cases are found to have fracture/dislocations, less than one-quarter fractures only, and a very small number are found to have involvement of the spinal cord with no obvious bony damage to the vertebral column, e.g. those with whiplash injuries. The most vulnerable areas of the vertebral column would appear to be:

lower cervical C_{5-7}
mid-thoracic T_{4-7}
thoraco-lumbar $T_{10}-L_2$.

The non-traumatic cases are mainly the result of transverse myelitis, tumours and vascular accidents. Thrombosis or haemorrhage of the anterior vertebral artery causes ischaemia of the cord with resulting paralysis.

Spinal cord damage resulting from either injury or disease may produce tetraplegia or paraplegia depending upon the level at which the damage has occurred.

Tetraplegia is partial or complete paralysis involving all four limbs and the trunk, including the respiratory muscles, as a result of damage to the cervical spinal cord.

Paraplegia is partial or complete paralysis of both lower limbs and all or part of the trunk as a result of damage to the thoracic or lumbar spinal cord or to the sacral roots.

Definition of the level of lesion

There are 30 segments in the spinal cord: 8 cervical, 12 thoracic, 5 lumbar and 5 sacral. As the spinal cord terminates opposite the first lumbar vertebra, there is a progressive discrepancy between spinal cord segments and vertebral body levels.

All cervical nerve roots pass through the intervertebral foramen adjacent to the vertebra of equivalent number. Roots C_1 to C_7 inclusive leave above the appropriate vertebral body, whereas root C_8 and the remainder exit below the appropriate vertebral body.

The higher the root, the more laterally it is situated within the spinal cord.

Although there is little difference between spinal cord segments and vertebral body levels in the cervical area, the nerve roots below C_8 travel increasing distances in the canal before exiting.

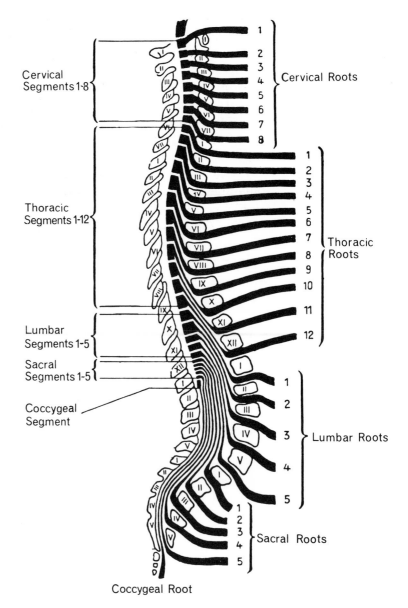

Cervical Segments 1-8

Cervical Roots

Thoracic Segments 1-12

Thoracic Roots

Lumbar Segments 1-5

Sacral Segments 1-5

Coccygeal Segment

Lumbar Roots

Sacral Roots

Coccygeal Root

Fig. 1.2 Topographical correlation between spinal cord segments and vertebral bodies, spinous processes, and intervertebral foramina. (From Haymaker W 1969 Bing's local diagnosis in neurological diseases, 15th edn. Mosby, St Louis.)

The 12 thoracic segments lie within the area covered by the upper 9 thoracic vertebrae, the 5 lumbar segments within that covered by T_{10} and T_{11} vertebrae and the 5 sacral segments lie within T_{12} and L_1 vertebrae.

There are several methods of classification of the level of lesion at present in use throughout the world. The system generally used in Great Britain is to give the most distal uninvolved segment of the cord together with the skeletel level, e.g. paraplegia, complete or incomplete below T_{11} due to fracture/dislocation of T_{9-10} vertebra (Fig. 1.2).

It may be described for instance as a transverse spinal cord syndrome, complete or incomplete below T_{11} due to fracture/dislocation of $T_{9/10}$. A lesion may not be the same on both sides, e.g. C_{5L}/C_{7R}. To give some idea of the neurological involvement in incomplete lesions, the most distal uninvolved segment is given together with the last segment transmitting *any* normal function, e.g. incomplete below C_5, complete below C_7. In this case some motor power or sensation supplied by C_6 and C_7 is present.

2

The team

TEAM WORK

The psychological reactions of the patient with spinal cord injury
present problems as formidable as the results of the disaster which
has suddenly reduced an individual in normal health and activity into
a state of complete immobility and dependence upon others. The full
psychological reaction to his physical condition inevitably develops
as the patient recovers from the initial traumatic shock. The reaction
will of course vary according to the intelligence, age and tempera-
ment of the individual.

To give maximum help to the patient during this period of
psychological readjustment as well as to achieve successful physical
rehabilitation, the team approach is essential. This can best be
achieved in a spinal injuries unit, where the individual patient lives
with others with the same disability and the various grades and
disciplines of staff are specifically trained. Besides gaining confidence from the expertise of the staff, the patient's contact with others
who are similarly affected but in the later stages of rehabilitation
provides visible evidence of what can be achieved.

At the centre of the team is the patient. In overall charge is the
director of the unit, who is the co-ordinator of the activities of the
individual medical and paramedical members of the team. He is
primarily responsible for the creation of the atmosphere of hope and
confidence in the success of the treatment so essential to the patient.
Team work according to the dictionary means 'co-operation' or 'to
make joint effort'. To work successfully in co-operation with others
demands general respect and understanding and an appreciation of
the work of the various disciplines. The expertise of each member of
the team is necessary if the needs of the 'whole man' are to be met.
The patient has been precipitated into an unknown and unreal world,
full of fears and problems. Only if he feels those around him are
vitally interested in his welfare and have expert help to give will he

regain confidence in himself. This confidence forms the basis of successful rehabilitation.

THE PHYSIOTHERAPIST–PATIENT RELATIONSHIP

Rehabilitation of the tetraplegic or paraplegic patient is a formidable and exacting undertaking for both patient and physiotherapist. For efficient rehabilitation in the shortest possible time there are two essential requirements:

1. The physiotherapist must know exactly what to ask the patient to do.
2. The patient must do exactly as he is asked.

The first depends upon the accurate knowledge and expertise of the physiotherapist, and the second depends primarily upon the confidence of the patient in the physiotherapist. Mutual confidence between the physiotherapist and the patient therefore plays a large part in successful rehabilitation. However, fear also plays a part in their reactions towards each other, and this must be overcome.
The patient fears, for example:

a. that he will not be able to do what he is asked to do.
b. that he will fall or injure himself.
c. that he is not going to get better or 'make the grade'.

The physiotherapist may fear:

a. that she will not know the right thing to say or do.
b. that she will not be able to answer the patient's questions.
c. that the patient will not do as she asks him.

Fear of failure is the keynote. From the earliest days of treatment the physiotherapist and patient must accept that they have a common objective and that their united efforts will result in progress, even though progress will be slow and variable. Without complete confidence, sympathy and co-operation between physiotherapist and patient, the prospect of success will be seriously prejudiced.
Confidence can be earned through concern and an honest approach and manner. The patient is, as a rule, acutely interested in his own condition, his reactions to treatment and his progress. It is essential that he shoud be given intelligible explanations of the treatment methods to be employed and agree the various long- and short-term goals for his therapy. He needs a reason for that which he is being asked to do and an understanding of how the present activity fits into the overall plan for his rehabilitation.
As the patient becomes progressively more independent, the

physiotherapist must also know when and how to gradually withdraw her support. It is essential that the physiotherapist remains tolerant and preserves an optimistic outlook in her dealings with the patient even though he may at times be querulous, fearful, complaining, lazy or disappointed.

3

Physiological effects and their initial management

CLINICAL EFFECTS OF SPINAL CORD INJURY

Severe injury to the vertebral column can occur from any direction and result in dislocation, fracture, or fracture/dislocation with or without resultant displacement. As a result, extensive trauma can occur to the spinal cord as it is compressed, crushed or stretched within the spinal canal (Hughes, 1984).

Yet there appears to be no absolute relationship between the severity of the damage to the vertebral column and that to the spinal cord and roots. A patient may sustain a severe fracture dislocation, and yet the spinal cord may be undamaged or only partially damaged. Another may exhibit no obvious vertebral damage on X-ray and yet have sustained an irreversibly complete tetraplegia.

The spinal cord not only conveys impulses to and from the brain but is also a nerve centre in itself, and through its various afferent and efferent pathways provides a vital link in the control of involuntary muscle. Transection of the cord will result in loss of

motor-power
deep and superficial sensation
vasomotor control
bladder and bowel control
sexual function.

At the actual level of the lesion there is complete destruction of the nerve cells, disruption of the reflex arc and flaccid paralysis of the muscles supplied from the destroyed segments of the spinal cord. This segmental reflex loss is of little importance when the lesion involves the mid-thoracic region, but when the cervical or lumbar enlargements are involved, some important muscles in the upper or lower limbs are inevitably affected with flaccid paralysis. In the same way a lesion at the level of the lumbar enlargement or cauda equina may destroy the reflex activity of the bladder and rectum and thus deprive the paraplegic not only of voluntary but also of involuntary (or automatic) control.

Lesions may be complete, where the damage is so extensive that no nerve impulses from the brain reach below the level of the lesion, or incomplete, where some or all of the nerves escape injury.

Immediately after injury the patient will be in a state of 'spinal shock'. The nerve cells in the spinal cord below the level of the lesions (i.e. the isolated cord) do not function. No reflexes are present and the limbs are entirely flaccid. This depression of nerve cell activity can last either a few hours or days in young people, or up to 6 weeks. Gradually the cells in the isolated cord recover independent function although no longer controlled by the brain. The reflexes return and the stage of spasticity ensues. As the spinal cord terminates at the level of the lower border of L_1, vertebral lesions below this level do not become spastic. The damage in these cases occurs to nerve roots only or is due to direct injury of the conus terminalis.

Occasionally a cord lesion of higher level may also remain flaccid. This is due to injury in the longitudinal as well as the transverse plane, or to longitudinal vascular damage.

Oedema or bleeding within the spinal cord may cause the level of the lesion to ascend one or even two segments within the first few days after injury. This is nearly always temporary, and the final neurological lesion will probably be the same or even lower than that found immediately after injury.

Spinal shock is not to be confused with the initial traumatic shock, which will certainly occur as with any other major trauma.

Associated injuries

Other skeletal or internal injuries may be present in addition to the spinal injury. Diagnosis of these injuries is rendered more difficult by the lack of sensation. The most common associated injuries are those of the long bones, head and chest. Head injuries are frequently found in conjunction with cervical fractures. Crush injuries of the chest with fractured ribs, pneumothorax or haemopneumothorax are commonly associated with fractures of the thoracic spine (Frankel, 1968). Abdominal injuries also occur in many cases.

Early complications

Chest complications

The paralysis of the muscles of respiration including the abdominal muscles can give rise to serious problems (see Ch. 5).

Deep venous thrombosis

Deep venous thrombosis, common between the 10th and 40th day post injury, is recognised clinically by characteristic swelling of the leg. Erythema and low grade temperature may also occur. Unless contra-indicated patients are given prophylactic anticoagulant therapy (Silver, 1975).

The swelling is frequently discovered by the physiotherapist when examining the limbs before giving passive movements. If a deep venous thrombosis is diagnosed in either one or both legs passive movements to both lower limbs are discontinued until the anti-coagulation has been stabilised.

Pulmonary embolism

This may occur within the first 2 or 3 months after injury. If an undiagnosed deep venous thrombosis is present, it may give rise to an embolus when the physiotherapist begins to move the leg. Many patients have pulmonary embolism without prior evidence of deep venous thrombosis.

Aims of treatment

A regime of treatment will be required for:

1. The initial traumatic shock.
2. Reduction and stabilisation of the fracture/dislocation.
3. The prevention of pressure sores and contractures.
4. The care of the paralysed bladder and bowels.
5. Physical and psychological rehabilitation.

POSTURAL REDUCTION

Various surgical procedures are used in some spinal injury units throughout the world to stabilise the fracture. In others and at the National Spinal Injuries Centre the initial treatment of the fracture/dislocation is conservative, that is, by postural reduction (Frankel, 1970; Guttmann, 1945, 1973).

Postural reduction is aimed at aligning the fractured vertebra and restoring and maintaining the normal curvature of the spine, though alignment of the vertebrae does not always imply recovery of the spinal cord.

After the initial X-rays are taken, pillows and/or a roll are used to place the spine in the optimum position to reduce the dislocation and allow healing of the fracture. The majority of injuries are the result of acute anterior or retroflexion of the spine, and the position has to be adjusted accordingly.

Control X-rays are taken over the next few days and weeks to check that the position is achieving the desired results. Plaster jackets or beds are *never* used because of the grave risk of pressure sores.

Fractured cervical spine

A firm small roll made of wool and covered with linen or tubegauze is used to support the fracture. This roll is placed on top of a single pillow which extends under the shoulders as well as under the head. (If further extension is needed a single pillow with the neck roll is placed under the head, and a double pillow, that is, two pillows in one slip, under the shoulders.) A double pillow is used to support the thorax and a single one is placed under the glutei and thighs with a 3-inch gap in between the pillows to prevent pressure on the sacrum. A pillow is placed underneath the lower legs to keep the heels off the bed and avoid pressure. A double pillow or several pillows bound together are set against the footboard to support the feet and toes in dorsiflexion.

If skull traction is necessary, and this is the case in the majority of cervical injuries, Cones Calipers are preferred and the weights are moderate, i.e. 6–15 lbs for 6 weeks on average.

Fractured thoracic or lumbar spine

A double pillow is usually sufficient to extend and support fractures of the dorsolumbar spine. Occasionally a third pillow may be necessary to obtain the correct degree of hyperextension.

Pillows have to be adjusted in such a way that the bony prominences are always free of pressure. The patient must be handled very carefully at all times. He must be lifted by four people or rolled in one piece with the fracture site well supported and the spine in correct alignment. Flexion and rotation particularly must be avoided.

Using this method of reduction, results are achieved which are better than those obtained through immediate surgery without any of the possible disadvantages of the latter. In particular there is less interference with the blood supply of the spinal cord, which may lead to further neurological damage. Occasionally a late surgical stabilisation procedure may be indicated where a cervical fracture remains unstable in both complete or incomplete lesions.

Correct positioning of the patient

Correct positioning of the patient in bed (see Ch. 5) is important in order:

    a. to obtain correct alignment of the fracture
    b. to prevent contractures
    c. to prevent pressure sores
    d. to inhibit the onset of severe spasticity.

Turning the patient

Patients are turned every 2 hours, day and night. The supine and side lying positions are used for the acute lesion. When using postural reduction the prone position is unsuitable. Once spinal shock has worn off 3 hourly turns are instituted and immediately prior to discharge home the time can be increased to 4 hours.

MANAGEMENT OF THE BLADDER

Disturbance of bladder function produces many complications which constitute a life-long threat to the patient. Statistics show that renal disease is responsible for the majority of deaths among patients with spinal lesions.

Assiduous and continuing bladder care is vital if complications are to be prevented.

Some relevant anatomical and physiological factors

The centre for micturition is located in the second and third lumbar and second, third and fourth sacral segments of the cord. It is linked to the detrusor muscle by parasympathetic, sensory and motor fibres which travel via the pelvic nerves.

The trigone and bladder neck are supplied by sympathetic motor fibres originating from spinal segments T_{11}–L_2. The external urethral sphincter and external anal sphincter are supplied by lower motor neurone fibres from S_2–S_4 and possibly also from L_5 and S_1.

The proprioceptors of the detrusor muscle respond to the increase of pressure as the bladder fills. Impulses travel via parasympathetic fibres to the sacral cord at S_2–S_4 and upwards through the spinothalamic tracts to the brain giving rise to the desire to void. The sensation that micturition is imminent originates in the urethra, and impulses reach the brain via the posterior columns.

Any lesion either above or involving cord segments T_{11}–S_4 will cause varying degrees of bladder dysfunction.

The acute lesion

The effect on the bladder depends upon the length of time after injury as well as the level of cord injury and the degree of cord damage.

Paralysis of the bladder during the first few days after acute spinal damage is total and flaccid. During this period of spinal shock all bladder reflexes and muscle action are abolished. The patient will develop acute retention, followed by passive incontinence due to overflow from the distended bladder.

Treatment will be directed to

— achieving a satisfactory method of emptying the bladder
— maintaining sterile urine
— enabling the patient to remain continent.

During the period of spinal shock, the bladder may be emptied in several ways including:

1. Urethral catheterisation
   a. intermittent
   b. indwelling.
2. Supra-pubic drainage.
3. Over distension therapy.
4. Electrical stimulation.

For acute lesions from whatever cause — traumatic, vascular, virus — the treatment of choice at the National Spinal Injuries Centre is intermittent catheterisation (Frankel 1984). This method allows some distension of the bladder which represents the physiological stimulus for micturition and triggers the appropriate impulses to the spinal bladder centre, thus promoting return of detrusor activity. An indwelling catheter leads to bladder infection.

Patients with total transection of the spinal cord no longer feel the specific sensations which indicate that the bladder needs emptying. Many patients, however, feel other sensations related to bladder filling and learn to interpret these as an indication that the bladder is full. The most common of the substitute sensations is a vague feeling of abdominal fullness which is the result of an increase in intravesical and/or intra-abdominal pressure.

Bladder training

As spinal shock wears off, which may take a few days to several weeks, two main types of bladder condition develop:

1. The automatic bladder.
2. The autonomous bladder.

The automatic (or reflex) bladder

This type of bladder develops in most patients with transverse spinal cord lesions above T_{10-11}.

As reflex tone returns to the detrusor muscle it contracts in response to a certain degree of filling pressure. The returning power of the sphincter is overcome and micturition occurs. This reflex detrusor action may be triggered off by stroking, kneading or rhythmic tapping over the abdominal wall above the symphysis pubis, or by stimulating other 'trigger' points, e.g. stroking the inner aspect of the thigh or pulling the pubic hair.

With training this reflex action will occur on stimulation of the 'trigger' points and not at other times, so that the patient can learn to empty his bladder every 2 or 3 hours and remain dry in between.

To express the automatic bladder in bed or on the toilet the patient taps the abdominal wall above the symphysis pubis with the ulnar border of one hand, or a clenched fist or with the tips of the extended fingers. The tapping is continued until micturition occurs. Tapping is then discontinued until the flow of urine ceases. This procedure is repeated until tapping fails to produce a contraction of the detrusor muscle.

Although tapping is found to be the trigger for many patients, others respond to different trigger points as already mentioned, or to a mixture of tapping and supra-pubic pressure.

The autonomous (or non-reflex) bladder

This bladder is virtually atonic and occurs where the reflex action is interrupted, that is, with a longitudinal lesion of the spinal cord or a lower motor neurone lesion. There is no reflex action of the detrusor muscle but the bladder can be emptied by supra-pubic manual pressure.

If the abdominal muscles are innervated the patient can raise the intra-abdominal pressure by straining, when the pressure on the kidneys is the same as that on the bladder. The disadvantage is that high pressure is also put on the rectum.

If the abdominal muscles are not innervated an external source of pressure is required. The disadvantage here is that the bladder pressure is raised above the kidney pressure.

To express this type of bladder in bed or on the toilet the patient places the clenched fist just above the symphysis pubis and pushes inwards and downwards leaning forward as he does so. The pressure is kept up until the flow of urine ceases. Several attempts will probably be necessary to empty the bladder.

Both the automatic and autonomous bladders may be emptied provided their function is understood, gradual training takes place and active infection of the bladder is avoided.

When out of bed the general increase in muscular activity,

especially of the abdominal muscles if innervated, may make it more difficult to keep dry. Consequently it may be necessary to express the bladder every hour at first.

Bladder training takes up a great deal of time and the patient may get discouraged, but it is important to persevere, for gradually the bladder will become trained and the time between the visits to the toilet lengthened to $1\frac{1}{2}$, 2, 3 and in some cases even 4 hours.

The same training is carried out for both sexes, but it is essential for the female patient as there is no satisfactory urinal at present on the market. Pads and rubber pants are the only protection in case of leakage between expressions. With encouragement, patience and perseverance this method is 60–65% successful among women, and it is well worth the effort involved.

Male urinals

There are several types of male urinals available. The best for any individual is that which he finds most convenient to use, but the following conditions must be fulfilled:

1. It must not cause pressure sores.
2. It must contain a non-return valve.
3. If not disposable, it must be easily cleaned and sterilised.

Condom type

The condom urinal is found to be the most satisfactory type for most patients. This consists of the condom, a nylon connector, a piece of rubber tubing and a bag for drainage (Fig. 3.1).

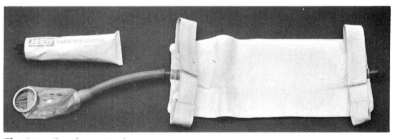

Fig. 3.1 Condum urinal.

Latex condoms are normally used. Nylon ones are available if the latex produces a skin reaction. The nylon connector is first placed inside the end of the condom and the connection tube is pushed over from the outside. This clamps the condom, which is then pierced where it stretches across the lumen of the connector. An orange stick is useful for this purpose. The shaft of the penis is smeared with suitable adhesive and the condom sheath is rolled on and held in place for at least 30 seconds to ensure that the glue becomes effective. The condom should extend at least 1 inch beyond the end of the penis. A finger stall may be more suitable than a condom for young boys. The connecting tube is then attached to the urine bag, which may be strapped to the leg when the patient is up, and hung from the frame of the bed at night. Disposable bags can be used or the more durable supra-pubic bag.

If the supra-pubic bag is used, each patient must have two and use them alternately so that each can be thoroughly disinfected after use. To disinfect the bag it should be washed in warm soapy water, rinsed, soaked in Dakin's solution (16%) for 2 hours, rinsed well and hung up to dry for 12–14 hours.

The Stoke Mandeville Hospital urinal and the Thackray male urinal

Both of these have a detachable penile sheath made in a number of sizes. As no adhesive is used this type is suitable for those patients whose skin reacts to the various adhesives used with the condom urinal. Both are bulky to use and more likely to cause pressure sores than the condom type.

Female pads

Incontinence pads and protective rubber or plastic pants are available from several manufacturers. Alternatively pads can be made up by the patient when size and thickness can be adjusted to suit individual needs — thin ones for use at home when the patient is in easy reach of the toilet, and thicker ones for travelling and visiting. The pads consist of 8-inch gauze tissue, white wool and cellulose tissue, and are approximately 5–6 inches wide and 12 inches long.

To make up the pad. Cut the wool and cellulose to the required size and the gauze tissue approximately 6 inches longer. Open out the gauze tissue on a flat surface and ensure that it is free from creases. Place the cellulose and the cotton wool, layered in that order, on to the gauze and fold the gauze over until the pad is completely enclosed. Tuck the end of the gauze neatly into the layers of wool.

The pad is worn with the white wool side next to the skin.

Urinary hygiene

All patients must be taught urinary hygiene to avoid smell and must learn to watch for skin abrasions, redness and septic spots. If damage to the skin on the penis occurs the urinal should not be worn until the lesion is fully healed. Severe pressure sores and fistulae can occur very rapidly if the urinal is applied over damaged skin. Difficult patches of adhesive may be removed with ether, but frequent use irritates the skin. Daily washing with soap and water and careful drying should be all that is required.

In order to have self-confidence the incontinent patient must be prepared to cope either alone or with minimal help at all times, not only at home but also when a suitable toilet may not be available. For the female patient, receivers or bedpans can be useful and expression of the bladder can be successfully carried out on a suitable bedpan in a wheelchair. The incontinent female patient will find it essential to have a small travelling case containing:

1. A plastic bedpan or receiver in a cover.
2. Clean pads.
3. Several plastic bags to receive soiled pads.
4. One plastic container of water for cleansing.
5. Talcum powder.

Autonomic hyperreflexia

Autonomic hyperreflexia is a vascular reflex which can originate in any organ below the level of the lesion in a patient with a high lesion. The physiotherapist must be alert to recognise the symptoms of autonomic hyperreflexia which are an outburst of sweating, slow pulse, raised blood pressure and headache. Overdistension of the bladder caused by a blocked catheter can give rise to this reflex activity which presents quickly and if not dealt with immediately can rapidly precipitate cerebrovascular accident, epileptic fits and even death. The treatment is to remove the cause. Drugs can be given as a temporary measure. Tilting the head up will reduce the blood pressure until further treatment can be given. Three cases of autonomic hyperreflexia were reported in the USA in 1980 which were precipitated by passive hip flexion. This occurred in young men with lesions at C_5, C_6 and T_1. It was suggested that this response was evoked by stretching the hip joint capsule or proximal leg muscles innervated by L_4, L_5 and S_1. (Mc Garry, 1982).

Caution *Should the symptoms of autonomic hyperreflexia occur when a patient is in the physiotherapy department prompt action should be taken.*

Sacral anterior root stimulators

Research continues on the use of sacral anterior root stimulators for bladder control. Radio linked implants have been successfully used to stimulate S_2, S_3 and S_4. By activating these the patient can empty the bladder at will. Initial results are encouraging (Brindley, 1984).

MANAGEMENT OF THE BOWELS

Immediately after the onset of paralysis fluids only are given because of the danger of a paralytic ileus of neurogenic origin. The bowel training regime is instituted once the patient is on a full diet.

Bowel training

The aim is to deliver the bowel contents to the rectum at the same time either daily or every second day and remove them by reflex defaecation when the patient is prepared for it. This is achieved by:

1. Mild aperients in the evening, e.g. 30 ml Sennocot granules.
2. Two glycerine suppositories the following morning followed half-an-hour later by digital evacuation with a gloved finger.
3. Correct diet and fluids.

Evacuation in bed

The previous evening Sennocot granules are given, 30 ml or as necessary depending on the results.

The following morning the patient is put on his left side and supported with sand bangs and pillows. A plastic sheet and one or two disposable incontinence pads are placed under the buttocks. Two glycerine suppositories are inserted into the rectum as high as the gloved finger can reach. Care is taken to avoid overstretching the anus or damaging the rectal mucosa. The patient is kept warm and given a hot drink. The rectum will empty itself is 20 or 30 minutes. It is advisable then to insert a gloved finger into the rectum to ensure complete emptying. The anus contracts when the finger is inserted. It then relaxes and the bowel empties.

Toilet training

When the patient is out of bed he is taught to do his own evacuation on the toilet once he has sufficient balance in sitting and is able to transfer with assistance. A bar is needed beside the toilet so that the patient can support himself whilst leaning forwards.

When the patient is upright, digital stimulation may no longer be necessary. Aperients and/or suppositories are continued as required.

The development of a regular habit of bowel opening is essential and with patience and perseverance it is possible to establish a satisfactory programme for all patients.

Tetraplegic patients continue manual evacuations on the bed unless they can get onto a commode or toilet chair. Prior to discharge the relatives or the district nurse are instructed in the procedure.

A patient with acute constipation may present with spurious diarrhoea, the impacted faeces allowing only liquids to pass through the gut. Although enemeta as a routine are avoided, in this case enemas may be given before starting the bowel regime.

SEXUAL DYSFUNCTION

Male

Male patients with high lesions often have priapism for hours or several days after injury. Subsequently all sexual function is abolished during the stage of spinal shock. Later return of function will depend upon the level and completeness of the lesion. For patients with complete lesions above the reflex centre in the conus automatic erections occur in response to local stimuli, but there will be no sensation during sexual intercourse. Patients with low cord lesions above the sacral reflex centres may not only have reflex erections but also psychogenic erections, if the sympathetic pathways are intact. Occasionally these may be accompanied by ejaculation. The seminal fluid will pass through the urethra only if there is an associated contraction of the internal bladder sphincter. Otherwise it refluxes into the bladder.

Reflex seminal ejaculation is rare in patients with complete lesions below T_{12}–L_1.

Sexual function varies widely in patients with incomplete lesions, according to the degree of cord damage sustained. Any form of sensation on the penis may indicate some preservation of genital sex. Problems may remain in relation to locomotor and voluntary muscle activity.

Tests can be carried out to assess potency and fertility (Guttmann, 1973).

Female

Menstruation

Interruption of the menstrual cycle occurs in the majority of women with complete or incomplete lesions who are not taking contraceptive pills. This can last from a few months to more than a year. Eventually the menstrual cycle returns to normal.

Pregnancy

Apart from lacking genital sensation sexual function is unimpaired for female patients with complete lesions.

Both paraplegic and tetraplegic women can become pregnant and have normal babies. These can be delivered vaginally or by caeserean section if indicated. Uterine contractions occur normally and because of the loss of sensation patients with complete lesions above T_{10} may have a painless delivery. Even patients with lower lesions may not be aware that labour has commenced, especially if it occurs during sleep. Therefore these patients should be kept under careful observation and are usually admitted to hospital before the expected delivery date.

PSYCHOLOGICAL CONDITION

Severe psychological shock must occur when a healthy, vigorous person is suddenly changed into a helpless invalid, utterly dependent upon others.

Initially the patient is too dazed to understand his condition. This period of initial shock may be prolonged when there is anoxia due to respiratory dysfunction or an associated head injury. Within a day or two in most cases, the patient becomes superficially aware of his disability. This knowledge gradually deepens and the patient begins to realise what the loss of movement and bladder, bowel and sexual function will mean in daily life. Uncertainty, fear and anxiety give rise to questions:

'Is this going to be permanent?'
'Will I ever walk or work again?'

The extent of the disability is forcefully brought home to the patient when he begins his rehabilitation in the wheelchair. During the acute phase in bed others cared for the body, but once up, the patient is confronted by his dependent, heavy, useless limbs. Many patients pass through a period of depression at this time. A more positive attitude usually develops as the day becomes filled with work and even slight progress is made towards independence.

Being amongst others in a similar plight helps the patient to realise the permanence of his disability and to adjust to the situation.

Depression may show itself in aggression to the staff or in antisocial behaviour. Patients more acutely depressed may develop various kinds of physical complaints including pain. This can become a fixation and can virtually stop further progress in rehabilitation. Others cannot face the reality of their problem and constantly affirm that they will walk again. In view of this they refuse to learn the activities of daily living from a wheelchair or to consider any necessary alterations to the home. A few, and perhaps the most difficult group, appear completely indifferent. They conform but are entirely apathetic.

In any spinal unit there is a wide variety of patients with as wide a variety of psychological make-up. Some patients have a long psychiatric history prior to admission, others sustain their injury attempting to take their own lives. These patients present particular problems and are obviously in need of special care.

All members of the rehabilitation team are concerned with the psychological readjustment of the patient. Each is responsible for his or her own contribution to the atmosphere of hope and confidence in which the patient can most easily come to grips with his disability. The relationship between the patient and individual members of the team must be one of confidence if the patient is to feel free to discuss his problems, and thus dispel some of his anxieties and frustrations.

It is important that the patient becomes aware not only of his potential in physical achievements but also of the limitations imposed by his disability. Only then will he develop a realistic attitude and be able to make the most of his rehabilitation and his talents and once again take up the responsibilities of home and family life.

A second period of depression may occur when the patient goes home, sometimes for the first weekend, often on discharge. From a sheltered life amongst others in wheelchairs, the patient is transferred into the hurly-burly of the able-bodied world where he may be stared at, ignored or even treated as a freak. In consequence there may be an initial tendency to shun social contacts until this barrier is overcome. Strong encouragement is needed from family or friends to go out and take part in social activities.

Not only the patient but the relatives also need to adjust to the situation. They too need to have a clear understanding of the patient's disability and what it will mean in home life.

Psychologists and sociologists suggest, and experience proves that the family provides the most effective link in the re-integration of the paraplegic or tetraplegic patient with his social environment (Ray, 1984).

Many spinal units provide an educational programme for those patients, relatives and friends who wish to take advantage of it (Houston, 1984).

The aim of the programme is to assist the members of the patients' family to understand what has happened and to give them the knowledge they need to take part in the process of rehabilitation (Pachalski, 1984). Subjects covered may include relevant anatomy, bladder and bowel function, spasm, skin care, sex and human relationships, aids and adaptations in the home, and employment.

In addition to instruction on patient care, the relatives need constant help, counsel and support by the staff. It is difficult to guard against being overprotective, but the relatives must be realistic about what the patient can do for himself and know how and when to give any assistance he may still require.

Communication between the patient and his family needs to be encouraged, as patients and relatives will often talk freely about the deeper issues involved with everyone except each other.

4

Important physical factors influencing the restoration of independence

The ultimate aim of rehabilitation is the restoration of independence. Many factors influence the degree of independence achieved such as the motivation of the patient, the skill of the therapist and the interaction of personality between patient and therapist, as well as the physical factors involved.

As with all patients, age and sex play a part in successful rehabilitation. The majority of patients incurring injuries to the spinal cord are young males, therefore expectations for the achievement of independence should be high.

Previous employment and leisure activities inevitably affect the existing strength of shoulder and shoulder girdle muscles. A coal miner will have greater strength in the shoulders and be more used to using his muscles than an office worker. Similarly, a trained athlete, horseman or squash player has greater co-ordination and visuospatial appreciation than a patient who has never used his body in these ways.

Three of the most important physical factors influencing the restoration of independence are the degree of motor function, the physical proportions of the patient and the amount of spasticity present.

MOTOR FUNCTION

The degree of motor function, which depends upon the level of the lesion, is obviously a crucial factor in determining the independence finally achieved. There is still much controversy among experts regarding the segmental supply of muscles, and the clinical examination of patients with spinal cord injury provides a fascinating study in this respect. An easy reference guide to the major segmental innervation of the most important muscles of the upper and lower limbs as described in *Gray's Anatomy* (35th edition) is provided in Appendix 1 and Appendix 2.

A rough guide to the amount of functional control of the joints of the upper and lower limbs at different segmental levels is given in Appendix 3.

A chart of progressive attainment in the 4 broad areas of daily living activities — self-care, wheelchair manoeuvres, transfers and gait — is given in Appendix 4. Each activity is listed at the highest segmental level at which it is currently attainable.

The segmental innervation of the skin

The approximate major dermatome levels on the anterior aspect of the skin of the trunk are:

Nipple line	T_5
Lower costal margin	T_7
Umbilicus	T_{10}
Groin	T_{12}
Genital and saddle areas	$S_{3, 4, 5}$

The segmental innervation of the skin of the arm and the leg are shown in Appendix 5.

PHYSICAL PROPORTIONS OF THE PATIENT

The physical proportions of the patient influence the ease and speed with which independence can be achieved.

Survey of patients with lesions at C_6

One of the most interesting developments in the rehabilitation of patients with spinal cord injury over the past 15 years has been the increasing degree of independence demanded from, and achieved by, patients with complete lesions of the cervical spine. The possibility of a tetraplegic patient *without* triceps, or with triceps of minimal strength, transferring from his wheelchair *unaided* or dressing either partially or independently, used not even to be considered, much less planned for in the rehabilitation programme. The most intrepid patients having led the way, therapists have gradually come to accept a greater degree of independence, particularly for patients with lesions complete below C_6.

Achieving this increased independence is expensive in effort and time for both the patient and the therapist and incurs extended hospitalisation. In 1977 a survey was undertaken at the National

Spinal Injuries Unit to look at the outcome of treatment in relation to two activities of daily living particularly difficult for patients with lesions at this level: the ability to transfer and the ability to dress. The group was restricted to those patients with a transverse spinal cord syndrome complete below C_6 where extensor carpi radialis was present and the triceps muscles was *absent* or graded 2 or less on the Oxford Scale.

The relevant data was extracted from the physiotherapy and occupational therapy records of 72 patients. The information required was not avilable for 6 of the patients, thus reducing the group to 66.

Transfers

To lift without triceps the patient must have a strong deltoid to hold the shoulder joint in three planes, an elbow joint capable of being locked in hyperextension and sufficient mobility in the wrist joint to allow weight to go through the arm with the palm on a flat surface.

As described in Chapter 11, transfers can be divided into three categories in order of difficulty, patients normally being taught the transfers in Group 1 first and progressing to those in Groups II and III where possible. For the purposes of the study:

Group I   included transfer chair ⟷ bed
chair ⟷ car
Group II included transfer chair ⟷ toilet
Group III included transfer chair ⟷ bath

The car transfer essentially lies between Groups I and II as the feet are raised to the horizontal in transfers in Group I and remain on the ground in those in Group II.

The results of the survey in relation to transfers are shown in Table 4.1. It is a ladder of progresssive attainment for the patient and does not indicate the ability to perform four random tasks.

Table 4.1 Transfers

	No. of patients	% of total
Unable to transfer	26	39
Bed only	23	35
Bed + car	11	17
Bed + car + toilet	4	6
Bed + car + toilet + bath	2	3

61% of the group were able to do some or all of the transfers. 35% transferred to the bed only.

26% could perform more than one transfer.

7 patients used a sliding board to transfer to the bed.

6 patients used a sliding board to transfer to the car.

Dressing

For descriptive purposes, dressing is divided into three sections (see Ch. 7): upper half, lower half and independent dressing.

Independent dressing for patients at this level of disability requires good balance unsupported in the sitting position, the ability to sit up from lying down and to roll from side to side. Extreme mobility in flexion at the hip joints is also necessary as the patient needs not only to be able to reach his feet when sitting with the legs extended, but to manipulate the clothing over the feet without hand and finger movement.

The results of teaching patients to dress are shown in Table 4.2. Patients were trained to do these tasks in the order shown: that is in the order of progressive difficulty.

Table 4.2 Dressing

	No. of patients	% of total
Unable to dress	8	12
Upper half only	33	50
Lower half with minimal help	16	24
Independent	9	14

Minimal help means assistance to pull the trousers over the hips and to put on the shoes.

88% of the group were able to dress the upper half.

38% could dress most or all of the lower half as well as the upper half.

It is highly significant that only 61% of the group were able to transfer whereas 88% were able to dress.

Sex distribution

Although these figures are not statistically significant, Table 4.3 shows the relative degree of success achieved by either sex. Motivation for dressing may be stronger in the women; all but one of the group were able to dress the upper half unaided but protective clothing for incontinence makes lower half dressing more difficult for women and none of the group was able to dress the lower half unaided.

Table 4.3 Degree of success achieved by either sex

	Men (49)		Women (17)	
	No. of patients	% of total	No. of patients	% of total
Able to transfer	34	69	6	35
Able to dress	42	86	16	94

It is interesting that no one lacked the motivation to learn all those tasks which are easier to achieve at this level of disability; for example, to wash, shave, clean the teeth and brush the hair.

The transfer depends upon the patient's ability to lift the weight of the trunk on the arms and this depends upon the strength of the shoulder muscles. Men have the advantage in this respect as in general they have greater strength in the shoulder girdle and have broader shoulders and narrower hips. Women by comparison have broad hips and are generally 'bottom heavy'.

Age

The age of the patients ranged from 12–61 years. Age did not appear to be a significant factor in this small sample, where 94% of patients were under 40 years old of these, 85% were under 30 years old. Some patients at the upper limits of the age range were able to transfer while some teenagers were not.

This survey showed that 60% of patients with lesions complete below C_6 can benefit from training in transfer techniques without using equipment, except for a sliding board, and 88% can benefit from training in dressing skills.

Height, weight and the length of the arms in relation to the length of the trunk appear to affect the rehabilitation of all patients with spinal cord injury, but particularly perhaps those with lesions complete below C_6.

In order to identify those patients most likely to benefit from extended rehabilitation it is necessary to determine the factors which differentiate between the successful and unsuccessful groups.

Physical ability in relation to anthropometric measurements in persons with lesions at C_6

A study was undertaken at the National Spinal Injuries Centre in 1981 (Berstrom et al) to assess which anatomical and anthropometric characteristics of the patient with tetraplegia complete below C_6

could be of value in predicting which patients would learn to transfer independently.

The same criteria were used in selecting the 36 chronic patients as in the survey described above. There were 33 males and 3 females and the ages ranged from 18–52 years. 23 anatomical and anthropometric variables were selected in order to give as complete a picture of the patient as possible. Spasticity, although difficult to quantify was included, as it was felt that, if severe, it could prevent patients from transferring independently.

Two groups of patients were defined: those who could transfer independently from a wheelchair to a surface of similar height (T) and those who could not (NT).

Table 4.4 shows the results for the total group of 36 patients, and for the subgroups representing Transfer and Non-transfer ability.

It is interesting that the data does not show the 'monkey-syndrome' (long arms and a short trunk) to be statistically significant for the ability to lift, although this is the subjective impression of therapists working in this field. Although not significant, functional arm length was greater in the Transfer group.

The largest significant difference between the two groups was in the base triangular measurement. This measurement was devised to get an impression of how much the subject leans forward in sitting and lifting (Fig. 4.1).

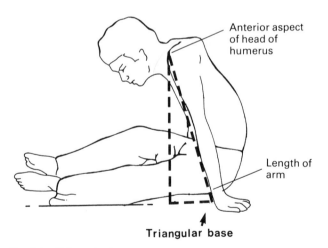

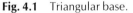

Fig. 4.1 Triangular base.

The 'triangle' was formed between:

a. the perpendicular from the anterior aspect of the head of the humerus
b. the distance along the floor to the hand
c. the length of the arm.

Table 4.4 Means and standard deviations of all the measured and predictor variables for the total group and the sub groups. The student's 't' value and its level of significance for the difference between Non-transfer and Transfer ability groups are also shown.

Variables	Units	Total group N = 36		Ability (Non-transfer) N = 25		Ability (Transfer) N = 11		t-value	Level of significance
		X̄	SD	X̄	SD	X̄	SD		
Age	a	28.4	7.9	29.1	9.0	26.7	4.8	1.0	ns
Weight	kg	65.7	14.3	68.4	15.0	59.6	11.0	2.0	ns
Stature	cm	176.1	9.2	176.3	9.3	175.5	9.4	0.2	ns
Sitting height	cm	93.1	4.5	93.4	4.3	92.2	5.0	0.7	ns
Cervicale to datum	cm	66.3	3.6	66.6	3.3	65.8	4.2	0.5	ns
Right shoulder flex	cm	10.6	1.8	10.3	1.6	11.1	2.1	1.1	ns
Left shoulder flex	cm	9.9	1.7	9.7	1.5	10.5	1.9	1.3	ns
Biacromial width	cm	38.5	2.5	38.4	2.5	38.9	2.6	0.6	ns
Bitrochanteric width	cm	34.4	2.4	38.8	2.1	33.5	2.7	1.4	ns
Functional armlength	cm	60.6	3.8	60.3	3.4	61.1	4.5	0.5	ns
Acromion to floor static	cm	59.0	4.2	59.1	3.5	58.8	5.7	0.2	ns
Acromion to floor lifting	cm	59.0	3.9	59.2	3.4	58.4	4.9	0.5	ns
Triangular base static	cm	12.5	5.6	11.6	4.0	14.4	8.1	−1.1	ns
Triangular base lifting	cm	13.0	5.4	11.0	4.3	17.1	5.4	−3.3	p<0.005
Head circumference	cm	57.9	1.8	57.8	1.8	58.1	1.8	−0.4	ns
Spasticity	grade	4.6	0.6	4.5	0.7	4.7	0.4	−1.3	ns
Σ4—skinfolds	mm	44.1	23.4	50.3	25.1	30.0	9.3	3.5	p<0.001
Fat % of body weight	%	17.9	6.6	20.1	6.3	12.9	4.1	4.1	p<0.001
Fat mass	kg	12.3	6.5	14.2	6.7	8.0	3.5	3.6	p<0.001
Fat free mass	kg	53.4	9.4	54.2	10.0	51.6	8.2	0.8	ns
Functional armlength/stature	cm	0.3	0.01	0.3	0.01	0.3	0.01	1.3	ns
Functional armlength/sitting height	cm	0.7	0.03	0.6	0.03	0.7	0.04	−1.4	ns
Functional armlength/cervicale to datum	cm	0.9	0.05	0.9	0.05	0.9	0.05	−1.3	ns

ns = not significant

The subjects with transfer ability leaned further forward when lifting. This gives greater mechanical advantage as it balances the body more accurately over the acromial point which is the fulcrum for the lift.

There was a significant difference between the two groups in the data on total body fat. This indicates that additional weight as fat is detrimental when attempting to lift and transfer.

The Non-transfer group had considerably broader hips. This forces the subject to place the arms further away from the sides, which effectively reduces arm length and minimises any mechanical advantage.

Morphologically females have narrower shoulders and broader hips than males. This data confirms the clinical impression that tetraplegic women do not lift as well as men and fewer can transfer.

As 23 variables were considered to be too many for practical use, an analysis was carried out on these variables to assess the extent to which a smaller number of anatomical and anthropometric data could predict the final ability to transfer.

Nine variables were finally selected:

1. biacromial width
2. body weight
3. cervicale to datum
4. fat %
5. head circumference
6. shoulder flexibility
7. sitting height
8. spasticity
9. triangular base lifting.

Using these variables it is possible to predict into which group (T or NT) a patient will fall with an accuracy of 90%.

However this result is tentative due to the small size of the sample. Data needs to be collected from a further sample of patients, and the present results used to classify patients into the Transfer or Non-transfer group, to assess the validity of the process.

SPASTICITY

There is no doubt that severe spasticity is one of the most inapacitating complications of spinal cord injury and can seriously curb rehabilitation, in some cases preventing even a minimal degree of self care. Early positioning of acute lesions has a great influence on the development of reflex patterns of spasticity in both complete and incomplete lesions. With adequate early treatment, the majority of patients are left with a degree of spasticity which is useful to them in many ways and which does not inhibit daily life. Some patients, however, develop incapacitating spasticity in spite of treatment.

The problems arising from severe spasticity are dealt with in the relevant sections of subsequent chapters.

5

Physiotherapy for the acute lesion

EXAMINATION OF THE PATIENT

For the therapist to gain maximum information regarding the patient she should be present at the initial neurological examination by the doctor in charge of the case.

In this way she will gain information regarding:

M.D.
1. the patient's injury
2. general condition
3. the site and condition of the fracture, if any
4. the presence of associated fractures or injuries, including any skin lesions
5. condition of the chest including the results of lung function tests
6. motor function
7. sensory function
8. presence or absence of reflexes
9. previous medical history
10. occupation
11. family history
12. diagnosis of the level of the lesion
13. immediate medical treatment.

The therapist will subsequently wish to make her own examination adding to the above information her assessment of:

P.T.
1. respiratory function
2. the range of motion of all joints involved and the presence of contractures
3. the strength of innervated muscles with particular regard to:
   —completely paralysed muscles
   —unopposed innervated muscle groups
   —imbalance of muscle groups.

4. the degree of spasticity, if present
5. the presence of oedema.

When the doctor and therapist discuss the treatment required, such factors as the following will be given special attention:

1. chest therapy, especially in relation to the treatment of patients on ventilators.
2. the danger of muscle shortening due to unopposed muscle action and the required positioning of the joints involved.
3. severe spasticity and the positioning required to gain relaxation.
4. the necessity for splinting.

After her own initial assessment the physiotherapist will need to discuss the case with the occupational therapist and the medical social worker.

Occupational therapy

All cases are seen by the occupational therapist but those with high cervical lesions will not need her skills at this early stage. Paraplegic patients are encouraged to do some form of work with their hands whilst in bed. Patients with cervical lesions with some hand or wrist function will be treated within a few days, that is, as soon as the period of traumatic shock is over.

Although assessment of the final outcome will be impossible at this early stage the medical social worker and the therapist work closely together from the commencement of the patient's stay in hospital.

Physiotherapy records

Detailed records are kept of the initial assessment, treatment and progress of the patient. Everyday incidents are also noted, such as the occurrence of bladder infections, slight injury or pressure marks, the first outing, and the first week-end home.

TREATMENT OF THE PATIENT IN BED

The patient with a spinal fracture will be in bed from 6–12 weeks. Those paralysed from other causes will spend considerably less time in bed.

Correct positioning of the patient

Correct positioning in bed is vitally important not only to maintain the correct alignment of the fracture, but to prevent pressure sores (p. 57) and contractures and to inhibit the onset of extreme spasticity.

The Supine Position (Fig. 5.1a)

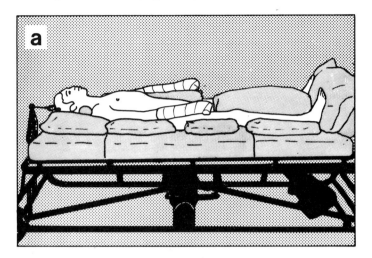

Fig. 5.1a Supine position of patient with a cervical fracture. (Right arm pillow was removed for clarity.) The patient is lying on an Egerton-Stoke Mandeville Electric Turning Bed.

When he is supine, the patient is positioned in the following way:

Lower limbs

    Hips   Extended and slightly abducted.
    Knees   Extended but not hyperextended.
    Ankles   Dorsiflexed.
    Toes   Extended.

One or two pillows are kept between the legs to maintain abduction and prevent pressure on the bony points, i.e. medial condyles and malleolli.

Upper limbs for patients with tetraplegia

    Shoulders   Adducted and in mid-position or protracted, but not retracted.
    Elbows   Extended; this is particularly important when biceps is innervated and triceps paralysed. If biceps is over-active, extension can be maintained by wrapping a pillow round the forearms, or by using a vacuum splint.
    Wrists   Dorsiflexed to approximately 45°.
    Fingers   Slightly flexed.

> *Thumb*   Opposed to prevent the development of a 'monkey' hand, which is functionally useless.

The arms are placed on pillows at the sides. The pillows should be high enough under the shoulders to ensure that the shoulders are *not* retracted. If the shoulders are painful and protraction is required, a small sorbo wedge can be placed behind the joint on either or both sides. If necessary two pillows should be used under the forearms and hands, as it is important that the hands are kept higher than the shoulders to prevent gravitational swelling in the static limbs.

The Side Lying or Lateral Position (Fig. 5.1b)

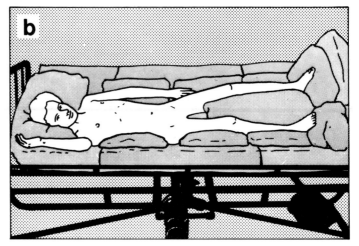

Fig. 5.1b Lateral position of patient with a low thoracic fracture.

When on his side, the patient is positioned in the following manner:

Lower limbs

Hips and knees	Flexed sufficiently to obtain stability with a double pillow between the legs and with the upper leg lying slightly behind the lower one.
Ankles	Dorsiflexed.
Toes	Extended.

Upper limbs

Lower arm	Shoulder flexed and lying in the trough between the pillows supporting the head and thorax to relieve pressure on the shoulder.
Elbow	Extended.
Forearm	Supinated and supported by a pillow on a table.
Upper arm	As in the supine position but with a pillow between the arm and the chest wall.

The Hand

If the hand is to be functional even when paralysed the maintenance of a good position in the acute phase is essential. The hand must remain mobile as it will be used in different positions, flat for transfers and flexed for all gripping movements as described on page 53.

Gravitational swelling must be avoided. If it is allowed to occur unchecked contractures easily develop.

Dr Cheshire (1970–1971) maintains that swelling can be prevented if the collateral ligaments of the metacarpophalangeal joints are kept at their maximum tension, i.e. when the joint is kept in 90° flexion. In order to prevent swelling and maintain a good functional position Dr Cheshire has developed the Boxing Glove splint (Fig. 5.2).

It consists of a light, well-padded, cock-up splint and a palmar roll. The wrist is maintained at 45° dorsiflexion, metacarpophalangeal joints at 90° flexion, interphalangeal joints at 30° flexion and the adductor web of the thumb in full stretch with opposition of the thumb. A layer of wool is placed over the dorsum of the hand and fingers and the whole bandaged as for an amputation.

The splint is removed several times a day for washing, physiotherapy and occupational therapy and the skin checked for pressure marks. It is used constantly for 8 weeks.

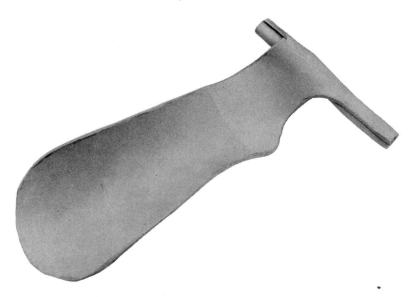

Fig. 5.2 Unpadded cock-up support for the Boxing Glove splint.

If the Boxing Glove splint is not used, the hand can be kept in a useful functional position by using a small palmar roll. Light straps keep the fingers in flexion and the thumb in opposition around the roll.

During the period in bed the following treatment is given:

1. Chest therapy—to maintain good ventilation.
2. Passive movements—to assist the circulation and to ensure full mobility of all paralysed structures.
3. Active movements—to maintain or regain muscle strength.

CHEST THERAPY

When the spinal cord is damaged, the respiratory muscles innervated below the level of the lesion become paralysed. This interferes with the power and integration of the remaining muscles and reduces their ability to drive the chest wall efficiently. Patients with injuries to the cervical spine have serious problems whilst those with lower thoracic and lumbar lesions have very little impairment of lung function.

All acute lesions need prophylactic chest therapy as all are subject to hypostatic pneumonia. The patient with partial or complete paralysis of any of the muscles of respiration will need special care.

The function of the normal chest wall and respiratory muscles

The current view of the action of the respiratory muscles on the chest wall is that an integrated activity of many muscles is probably required to expand the rib cage in the most efficient way.

The respiratory muscles comprise three main groups: the diaphragm, the intercostal/accessory muscles and the abdominal muscles. These muscles act upon the chest wall either as prime movers or to strengthen the rib cage and facilitate the action of the others.

Diaphragm: innervation C_4

The diaphragm is the major inspiratory muscle. It does not have an expiratory action. As the diaphragm contracts, the central tendon is pulled downwards and forwards pushing before it the abdominal viscera. It expands the rib cage using the abdominal viscera as a fulcrum. The product of diaphragmatic action will depend upon the balance of both rib cage and abdominal compliance. Consequently it will vary according to different conditions, for example with posture or spasticity.

Intercostal muscles: innervation T_1-T_7

The major action of the internal and external intercostal muscles is to stabilise the rib cage so that the diaphragm can act upon it. Both groups of muscles have an inspiratory action at low lung volumes and an expiratory action at high lung volumes.

Scaleni: innervation C_2–C_8

The scaleni muscles are now considered to be primary respiratory muscles. They lift, expand and stabilise the rib cage from their insertion on its upper part.

Accessory muscles of respiration: innervation C_2–C_4

In tetraplegia the sternomastoid ($C_{2,3}$) and trapezius ($C_{2,3,4}$) are the most important accessory muscles of respiration because of their high segmental supply.

The sternomastoid contributes to inspiration only during exercise or stress.

Abdominal muscles: innervation T_6–T_{12}

The abdominal muscles are muscles of expiration. Their action is to collapse the rib cage and force the diaphragm and abdominal contents up into the thorax to empty it from below. They are the most important muscles in *forced* expiration and participate vigorously in coughing, vomiting and defaecating.

They are inactive during quiet respiration, as gravity and the elastic recoil of the thoracic cage appear sufficient to produce expiration.

They provide an elastic wall to retain the viscera and to oppose the action of gravity on the viscera when standing or sitting.

Consequences of respiratory muscle paralysis

During the period of spinal shock when there is an absence of tone in all muscles below the level of the lesion, the distensibility of the rib cage and abdominal wall prevents the diaphragm from inflating the lungs in the most effective way. When the period of spinal shock is over and the reflexes return, the degree of tone in the intercostal muscles will, in general, improve the stability of the rib cage and also provide some resistance in the abdominal muscles, thus rendering the action of the diaphragm more effective (Guttmann 1965; Silver 1970).

The fall in vital capacity below the value that would be expected from the loss of motor power alone, and the rise which often occurs even in the absence of neuromuscular activity, reflect the distortion of the rib cage and its later improvement as tone returns to the intercostal muscles and the rib cage joints stiffen (De Troyer 1983; Morgan 1984).

Due to the paralysis of the respiratory muscles:

1. The patient is unable to perform active, expulsive expiration.
2. *Total* rib cage and lung inflation is impossible.
3. The partial loss of inspiratory muscle function allows the pleural pressure generated by the diaphragm to distort the rib cage which results in paradoxical motion. This can be seen in the absence of tone when the intercostal spaces are indrawn during inspiration.
4. This increases the work of breathing and reduces the effectiveness of the action of the diaphragm.
5. Without active abdominal muscles the patient is unable to cough.
6. The inability to inflate parts of the lung and to clear secretions tends to produce micro-atelectasis with subsequent fibrosis of lung tissue.
7. Small areas of collapse immediately after injury interfere with ventilation and may result in transient hypoxaemia.
8. The reduction in available muscle power and the increased load placed on the remaining muscles of respiration increases the likelihood of respiratory muscle fatigue and failure (Morgan, 1984).

Effect of posture

In the supine position the action of the diaphragm is assisted by the weight of the abdominal viscera displacing the diaphragm cranially and assisting inspiration. In sitting the abdomen may be so lax that the diaphragm has nothing to work on. Consequently there is a fall in vital capacity when the patient assumes the upright position. Research has shown that the vital capacity of the tetraplegic patient improves by 6% when the patient is tipped 15° head down from the supine position and falls by approximately the same amount when the head is tipped up 15°.

Methods of treatment

In view of the consequences of respiratory paralysis the aims of treatment are:

1. to increase lung volume
2. to clear secretions from the lungs.

Improvement in lung volume will:

a. increase the respiratory reserve at times of stress
b. assist in preventing atelectasis and lung fibrosis
c. increase the effectiveness of cough because the elastic recoil pressure increases with lung volume.

The vital capacity of patients with cervical lesions below C_4 falls to approximately 58% of normal and that of patients with high thoracic lesions to approximately 73% of normal. Where the abdominal muscles are paralysed the patient is unable to cough. All patients need chest therapy for at least the first 3 weeks post injury and some will require it until they get up.

In order to measure progress and keep a close watch for deterioration in those with respiratory muscle paralysis, the vital capacity should be measured and recorded before and after each treatment session. The physiotherapist should watch for any change in breathing pattern especially noting any rib cage paradox.

Breathing exercises

Inspiration

All patients need deep-breathing exercises to ensure good ventilation and increase the lung volume. Where possible localised diaphragmatic, lateral costal and apical breathing exercises are given.

In cases with lesions above T_1, where the diaphragm is the only muscle of respiration innervated, the vital capacity falls to between 700 ml and 1000 ml immediately after injury. The breathing is shallow and the hollow between the anterior costal margins rises only slightly with each inspiration. To encourage the patient to use the diaphragm the therapist gives light pressure with her hand just below the sternum. The position of the therapist's hand appears to assist the patient to concentrate on his diaphragm even where there is loss of sensation over the thoracic and abdominal walls. As the diaphragm becomes stronger the paralysis of the inter-costal muscles is more obvious, the intercostal spaces being drawn in at each inspiration. With the return of reflex activity to the isolated cord the intercostal muscles become spastic.

Expiration

During successive expirations the therapist gives pressure over the thorax with the hands spread as wide as possible. The position of the hands is changed after each breath until as much of the thorax as possible has been covered. This manipulation has a squeezing action on the thoracic cage. It produces a slightly *forced* expiration which is followed by a more efficient inspiration.

Intermittent positive pressure breathing

Intermittent positive pressure breathing and/or resisted inspiratory exercise training may increase lung expansion and therefore lung volume (Higgs). Research into these possibilities is being undertaken at the National Spinal Injuries Centre.

Assisted coughing

The patient with partial or complete paralysis of the abdominal muscles is incapable of cughing. To produce an effective cough the therapist's hands must replace the work of the abdominal muscles by creating pressure underneath the working diaphragm.

Methods of assisting the patient to cough

1. The hands are spread anteriorly around the lower rib cage and upper abdomen. The therapist pushes inwards and upwards as the patient tries to cough. The pressure is given evenly and firmly with the weight of the therapist's body behind the 'push'. The force required is difficult to gauge. It must not be sufficient to move the cervical spine or cause pain at the fracture site, but must deliver the sputum to the mouth. The sound of the cough produced is a good guide to the force needed. Jerky movements or pressure on the abdominal wall alone must be avoided, as a patient with an acute lesion may have a paralytic ileus or some as yet unknown internal damage (Fig. 5.3a and b).

Alternative positions for the hands are:

—on the lateral aspects of the thorax, with one forearm across the diaphragm and lower ribs.

—one hand on the upper sternum and the other over the diaphragm.

The last position is useful if the sputum is sticking high in the trachea.

Methods using two therapists

If the chest is infected and the sputum tenacious, or if the patient has a large thorax or easily becomes exhausted, one therapist may not be able to give the necessary pressure to produce a cough. In this case two therapists working together in one of the following ways usually proves effective.

1. Standing on either side of the bed the therapists place their forearms across the chest with the hands curved round the opposite side of the chest wall. The arms are placed alternately with the lowest arm across the diaphragm. When the patient attempts to cough the therapists squeeze the chest (Fig. 5.3c).

2. Standing on either side of the bed, each therapist spreads her hands over the upper and lower ribs of the same side with the fingers

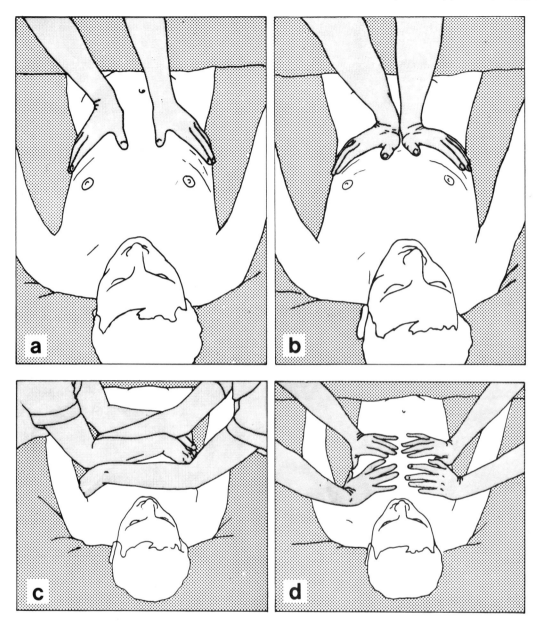

Fig. 5.3 Assisted coughing.

pointing towards the sternum. When the patient attempts to cough the therapists simultaneously push on the chest wall (Fig. 5.3d).

Frequency of treatment

It is important that the patient coughs several times a day to clear the throat even though the chest appears free from secretions. Patients with high lesions cannot clear the throat unaided, and the normal amount of debris delivered daily from the lungs collects in the upper trachea. Although this will not cause distress for the first 2 or 3 days, towards the end of a week the patient will begin to feel some difficulty in breathing. Inspiration becomes slightly laboured, and finally the debris is pushed down into the bronchial tree. At the end of the week a patient with a previously clear chest may suddenly develop a high temperature and be found to have pneumonia or collapse of a lung.

This can be prevented by prophylactic treatment given three or four times a day for the first 2 weeks at least. Treatment is subsequently given once a day until the patient is up in a wheelchair and able to clear his secretions unaided. Tetraplegic patients also need prophylactic postural drainage at least once a day. If a mobile cervical patient with a lesion at or above C_5 gets a heavy cold, he should return to bed for 24 hours. This prevents the nasal secretions dropping down into the chest and causing congestion. He will need assistance to blow the nose and clear the throat.

Treatment for the patient with an infected chest

Postural drainage

Unless contra-indicated, postural drainage may be given to any lesion to help clear secretions from the lungs. Care is taken to gain the correct drainage position for the area affected within the limits imposed by the hyperextended position and the type of bed in use.

With the patient in the correct position the following treatment is given:

1. Inspiratory exercise—localised breathing is given where possible using all innervated muscles.
2. Vibrations, shaking and percussion are given to help dislodge the sputum from the bronchial walls. Each series of vibrations is continued just beyond the extreme limit of expiration and terminates in firm pressure. The vibrations and shakings are given, during successive expirations, all over the chest wall and particularly over the affected area.

Caution Percussion is not given to patients with severe chest injuries. Very careful vibrations only are given in such cases.

3. Assisted coughing (see p. 40).

The drainage position is maintained for up to 20 minutes in the absence of contra-indications such as a heart lesion or head injury. As secretions easily move from one area to another in the paralysed chest, it will be necessary to drain the unaffected areas also. With experience, the therapist will be able to 'feel' abnormalities of air-entry with her hands on the chest wall as well as via the stethoscope and concentrate her treatment on these areas.

Frequency of treatment

The frequency of treatment depends upon the severity of the chest infection. 'Little and often' is a good maxim. If the patient tires quickly and has copious sputum it may be necessary to treat him every hour, day and hight for 24 hours. For less severe cases treatment every 2 hours, that is, at each turn will be sufficient. It is important to give postural drainage before as well as after the turn and essential when treating high lesions. If both lungs are congested and the uppermost lung is not cleared before the turn, as the patient is moved secretions may drain into the trachea completely blocking it and choking the patient. This can be prevented if the uppermost lung is cleared before the patient is moved. The therapist should wait whilst the patient is turned and treat him immediately in the new position, before the sputum has a chance to settle.

As the chest clears treatment is reduced accordingly. A patient on a ventilator needs regular postural drainage.

Mechanical ventilation

A patient may require mechanical ventilation for the following reasons:

1. If the lesion involves C_4 and the diaphragm is paralysed.

2. Owing to bleeding and oedema within the spinal canal, any lesion may rise by one or two segments during the first few days after injury. If this occurs when the lesion is at C_5 the diaphragm may cease to function.

3. If there are severe chest injuries a patient with a comparatively low lesion may need a ventilator to ensure that expansion is adequate and the fractures of the thoracic cage heal in a good position.

4. If there is a previous medical history of chronic chest disease.

Only if mechanical ventilation is necessary for longer than 2 weeks is a tracheostomy performed. For shorter periods intubation and intermittent positive pressure ventilation are used.

Tracheostomy is not considered necessary where the diaphragm is innervated but the chest infected. Constant physiotherapy day and night is usually sufficient to clear the chest. A tracheostomy may be considered, if the patient has a previous medical history of chronic bronchitis and emphysema and this has produced a rigid thorax.

Vital capacity

If the vital capacity falls to between 500–600 ml it is checked every half-hour. A further fall will probably indicate that mechanical assistance is necessary. The therapist should immediately report to the doctor any change in the patient's responses. Slower speech or an inability to co-operate in treatment because he falls asleep after the least exertion may mean that the patient is hypoxic.

Management of the tracheostomy

A tracheostomy reduces the respiratory 'dead space' by approximately one-half. In consequence each breath becomes more effective in oxygenating the blood and removing CO_2. It also facilitates the removal of secretions from the lungs and the control of oxygen administration. In the acute state a cuffed tracheal tube is commonly used as this provides an effective seal for the lungs against secretions or inhaled substances and will readily connect with the tube from a ventilator, should this be required.

The cuff

Overinflation of the cuff for long periods can cause excessive pressure on the tracheal mucosa and lead to necrosis, sloughing and stricture formation later. Excessive pressure is avoided by inflating the cuff just sufficiently to make the seal and by deflating the cuff at intervals for a short time. Oropharyngeal suction, preferably in the head-down position, is given before deflating the cuff, so that secretions do not run down into the lungs alongside the tube.

The tube is changed frequently as the lumen can become blocked by encrusted dried secretions.

Humidification

Some form of humidification will be necessary to warm and moisten the inspired air, which no longer passes through the nasopharynx. It is important to avoid hardening of the secretions and drying and possible trauma of the mucosa of the respiratory tract.

Suction

Tracheal suction should be carried out as often as is necessary to keep the airways free from secretions. This has to be done with great caution to avoid cardiopulmonary reflexes.

Equipment

A whistle-tipped suction catheter is used. This should not be larger than half the diameter of the tracheostomy tube. A larger catheter allows too great a negative pressure to develop in the lungs, which can cause gross plumonary congestion followed by sudden cardiac failure. The negative pressure should be as low as possible, consistent with the removal of the secretions. More powerful suction is required when the sputum is thick and tenacious.

Technique

To minimise infection a 'non-touch' technique is employed, the emphasis being on sterility, thoroughness and gentleness. Disposable gloves are used to guide the catheter into the tube. If preferred, forceps can be used in addition. Some sensitivity in handling the catheter and sucking out secretions is lost when using forceps, although they may add to the sterility of the procedure. Each sterile catheter is inserted once only before being discarded. The catheter is pinched whilst being introduced into the tube to allow suction only on withdrawal and prevent damage to the tracheal mucosa. Similarly, if the catheter is mounted on a Y piece, one end is left open whilst inserting the catheter. Death from cardiac arrest has been known to occur during suction. The underlying physiology is still obscure, but in view of the danger suction is maintained for only *10* seconds at a time. Maximum efficiency is obtained if the catheter is rotated slowly as it is withdrawn.

Management of a patient on a ventilator

The ventilator will be adjusted by the doctor in charge of the case according to the daily reports on the patient's blood gases. The therapist should familiarise herself with the particular type of ventilator in use and check with the doctor the rate and pressure at which the machine is to function. The therapist should also know how to measure the minute volume and how to use a spirometer to measure the vital capacity when the patient is disconnected from the ventilator. It is essential that the therapist and nursing staff attending the patient know how to switch the machine over from the mains electricity to battery supply in case of an electricity power cut or failure. An ambu bag should be kept beside the patient's bed with a tracheostomy connection, as well as a face mask, in case the ventilator breaks down completely.

Communication with the patient

To be nursed on a ventilator is a strange and terrifying experience for the patient. Understanding, cheerfulness and honesty are particularly important in the staff treating these cases. Electronic calling devices are available which allow patients with high lesions to operate the sensor either during mechanical ventilation or when breathing spontaneously. To avoid unnecessary distress the patient should be told exactly what is going to take place, and the ventilator should never be disconnected without first asking the patient if he is ready. As the inflated cuff prevents speech, it is important to devise some means of general communication. If initially unable to 'mouth' words adequately, the patient may be able to answer *yes* and *no* by using some facial expression such as blinking or winking. Later, he will learn to speak during *insufflation*, whilst the cuff is deflated.

Treatment

Postural drainage will be given regularly. The frequency of treatment will depend upon the condition of the chest and the quantity of secretions present.

After treating the patient on the ventilator, bag-squeezing may be employed to aid loosening of the sputum in the small bronchii and to increase expansion at the base of the lungs. The ventilator is disconnected and the patient inflated manually using repeated bag compression for not more than 3 minutes. The tracheostomy is then sucked out and the patient re-connected to the ventilator.

Caution *Bag-squeezing is contra-indicated if the patient has hypertension or a pneumothorax.*

If the diaphragm is totally paralysed and the patient unable to tolerate more than a few seconds without the ventilator, it is advisable for the therapist to have an assistant to suck out the trachea. When the assistant is ready, the therapist disconnects the ventilator. After the catheter has been inserted the therapist vibrates and shakes the chest whilst the assistant slowly withdraws the catheter, sucking out the secretions which are being squeezed into the bronchus. Immediately after the catheter is withdrawn, the therapist reattaches the ventilator.

The therapist should watch for signs of oxygen lack, i.e. cyanosis and sweating, restlessness, decreased level of consciousness, and report any changes to the doctor immediately.

If there is a loss of tidal volume:

1. There may be some obstruction in the tubes of the apparatus, i.e. water may have condensed in the hoses of the humidifier and formed a pool in a dependent loop.

2. Sputum may have accumulated. This can happen quite silently in quantities large enough to block the larger bronchii.

3. Bronchial spasm may be present. If bronchospasm is a problem it may be necessary to ask for a bronchodilator to be given before treatment, e.g. aminophilline by injection, isoprenaline administered via a nebuliser.

Weaning the patient off the ventilator

As soon as there is some return of function in the diaphragm the patient is disconnected from the ventilator for short periods several times a day. During these periods the therapist encourages the use of the diaphragm and the accessory muscles of respiration.

With systematic exercise the accessory muscles can be hypertrophied. Their action is particularly useful when the diaphragm remains partially paralysed.

Caution *In the early stages care must be taken during exercise to keep the head still and the neck extended.*

Initially the patient may only manage 30 seconds at a time off the ventilator. As the diaphragm gets stronger, longer periods are gradually achieved until the patient can remain without the ventilator during the day but is unable to sleep without it. It is usually fear that prevents sleep, and this is gradually overcome. During the weaning period, which may take several weeks, the patient needs a great deal of encouragement. He should be told exactly what to expect and be warned against being too disappointed when improvement is slow, or when there appears to be no improvement at all for a time.

The ventilator should be replaced whenever the patient asks for it, otherwise he becomes afraid of having it disconnected. This fear will slow down progress. After a moment or two, with encouragement the ventilator can usually be disconnected again. It is helpful to keep a chart of the time spent off the ventilator.

If the diaphragm is innervated and the ventilator is being used because of chest injuries, the weaning should take place within 3–7 days.

It is possible to place a cork in the tracheostomy tube for short periods to allow speech. When the cork is in place, the patient may complain of feeling unable to breathe, but again with encouragement and perseverance he will overcome his fear.

When the patient no longer needs the ventilator and the chest is sufficiently free of secretions, the tracheostomy tube will be changed for a smaller one with a speaking tube. With the stoma closed by the speaking tube assisted coughing will be possible. Gradually coughing replaces suction, the catheter only being used at the end of treatment to check that the coughing has been effective.

Diaphragmatic pacing using phrenic nerve stimulation

It is unusual for patients with injuries at C_1 and C_2, where all the muscles of respiration are paralysed, to survive until they reach hospital. In exceptional circumstances and occasionally if the lesion is incomplete, the patient survives to become totally dependent on a life support system. Until recently this meant the use of a ventilator, but the development of the phrenic nerve stimulator has given these patients a new independence (Collier 1982).

The stimulator is wrapped around one of the phrenic nerves in the neck. On the same side a radio frequency receiver is placed in a skin pocket fashioned over the 5th and 6th ribs. Electrode leads connect the stimulator and the receiver through a subcutaneous tunnel. The receiver is activated by a small transmitter attached to an antenna on the skin. A strain of gradually increasing electrical impulses brings about a smooth contraction of the diaphragm resulting in inspiration.

This is repeated on the other side so that each hemi-diaphragm has a separate stimulator. Training is started by pacing each side for only 5 minutes at a time to prevent muscle fatigue. This is increased slowly. The aim is to enable the patient to breathe via the stimulator initially during the day and for 24 hours if possible.

When there is trauma to the phrenic nerve the stimulator cannot be used. Similarly it is not used when the lesion involves $C_{3,4,5}$ because the phrenic nerve arises from these anterior roots.

Paralytic ileus

The initial signs of this complication, often first noticed by the physiotherapist, are distension of the abdomen and/or complaints by the patient of difficulty in breathing. This can be particularly dangerous for the tetraplegic patient with his already embarrassed respiration. If such a patient is likely to vomit he is turned from side to side only until the danger is passed.

2. PASSIVE MOVEMENTS

Passive movements of the paralysed limbs are essential to stimulate the circulation and preserve full range of movement in joints and soft tissues. Treatment is commenced the *first* day after injury. During the period of spinal shock, that is, for approximately 6 weeks, treatment is given twice daily. Movements are continued once a day until the patient is mobile and capable of ensuring full mobility through his own activities. Approximately 10 minutes are spent on the movement of each limb. A high proportion of this time is given to slowly moving the limb as a whole to improve the circulation.

In addition each joint starting proximally and working distally and including the metatarsal and metacarpal joints, is moved several times through its full range, and appropriate movements are given to prevent muscle shortening. The movements are performed slowly, smoothly and rhythmically to avoid injury to the insensitive, unprotected joints and paralysed structures. Any limitations imposed by previous medical history and/or age must be taken into consideration.

When reflex activity returns, the limb must be handled with extreme care, so as not to elicit spasm and reinforce the spastic pattern. A pinch grip or any sudden brisk movement must be avoided. If a spasm occurs during a movement the therapist holds the limb firmly and waits for the spasm to relax before completing the movement. Forced passive movements against spasticity may cause injury or even fracture of a limb. Sometimes, however, the only way to overcome ankle clonus is to *completely* dorsiflex the ankle, against the spasm, and hold it until the foot relaxes. The movement must be performed firmly but gently.

The importance of detail when giving passive movements cannot be overemphasised if the functional range in *all* structures is to be maintained.

Cautions

1. Extreme *range of movement must be avoided, particularly at the hip or knee, as the tearing of any structures may be a predisposing factor in the formation of para-articular ossification.*

2. *Only 45° abduction is given to avoid tearing any structures on the medial side of the thigh. The medial side of the knee must always be supported to prevent stretching the medial ligament.*

3. *Flexion of the hip with the knee flexed is cautiously carried out where there is a fracture of the lower thoracic or lumbar spine to ensure that movement does not occur in the lumbar spine. If pain occurs on movement, flexion is limited to the pain-free range. The range of movement is gradually increased as the pain at the fracture site diminishes. When the patient is supine, full flexion of the knee can only be obtained by combining knee flexion with lateral rotation of the hip.*

4. *Straight-leg raising is limited to 10° in all cases because of the danger of putting a stretch on the dura mater. Dorsiflexion of the*

ankle is given at the same time to increase the stretch of the hamstrings.

5. Combined flexion of the wrist and fingers is never given. This movement can cause trauma of the extensor tendons resulting in loss of mobility and function.

Maintenance of muscle length

Gross contractures occur when a paralysed limb is not moved, but contractures can occur also in individual muscles or muscle groups in a limb which is receiving daily treatment.

For example contractures readily occur in the following situations:

1. Where the muscle on one side of a joint is innervated and the opposing muscle paralysed.
2. Where a paralysed muscle passes over more than one joint, individual joint movements are insufficient to maintain the muscle length.
3. When the patient lies with the spine in hyperextension to heal a fracture. The degree of hyperextension necessary to correct fracture dislocations of the lower thoracic and lumbar spine inevitably produces slight flexion of the hip joints. In cases with fracture of the cervical spine the shoulders are held in elevation and retraction due to gravity and unopposed muscle pull.

For these reasons the movements mentioned in the following section must be given in *addition* to the full range of passive movements.

The shoulder girdle

Particular attention needs to be given to the shoulder girdle. It is so freely movable that its habitual position depends upon the relative tension in the following six muscles:

Trapezius	Cranial 11, C_3, C_4
Levator scapulae	C_3, C_4, C_5
Rhomboids	C_5
Serratus anterior	C_5, C_6, C_7
Pectoralis minor	C_8, T_1
Subclavius	C_5, C_6

together with the tension produced by

Pectoralis major	C_5, C_6
Latissimus dorsi	C_6, C_7, C_8

which act indirectly on the shoulder girdle through the arms. The mobility of the shoulder girdle is largely maintained through *adequate* unilateral and bilateral passive movements to the arms, which will prevent shortening of these muscles.

The scapula

Mobility of the scapula must be maintained. Movements are performed passively in lying or side lying with the elbow well supported by the therapist.

Passive depression is particularly important where the muscles of elevation are innervated and unopposed.

In situations where physiological or passive movements of the limbs are impractical, accessory gliding techniques should be applied locally to the joints involved to maintain mobility.

To prevent shortening of the:
Rhomboids

With the arms in horizontal flexion, adduct both shoulders at the same time. Both elbows are flexed and each hand moves towards the opposite shoulder.

Long head of triceps

With the arm held in elevation flex the elbow.

Pectoral muscles

Abduct and extend the shoulder, with the elbow, wrist and fingers extended and with the forearm supinated.

Biceps

Pronate and supinate the forearm with the elbow flexed *and* with the elbow extended. (Pronation is particularly important for patients with lesions at C_5 since biceps pulls the forearm into supination, and this is not a functional position.)

Flexor tendons of the fingers

Extend the wrist and fingers together.

Flexor muscles of the arm

Elevate and laterally rotate the arm with the forearm supinated, elbow, wrist and fingers extended and with the arm held close to the side of the head.

Hip flexors, quadriceps and anterior fascia of the thigh

In side lying extend the hip through the last 15° of movement keeping the knee flexed. The posterior aspect of the hip must be well supported to prevent movement occurring in the spine.

Tensor fascia lata

Adduct and medially rotate the leg beyond the midline.

Tendo-achilles

Dorsiflex the ankle with the knee extended.

Flexor muscles of the toes

Extend the toes, dorsiflex the ankle and extend the knee. Clawing of the toes occurs easily and not only hinders walking and increases spasticity but may lead to pressure sores on the dorsal and/or plantar aspect of the toes.

Careful attention must also be given to movements involving rotation and flexion of the limb. For example, flexion and lateral rotation of the hip with flexion of the knee are important for self-dressing.

Inspection of the lower limbs

Before commencing treatment the therapist examines the legs for signs of swelling or pressure. Deep vein thrombosis is a common complication during the early weeks after injury, and the possibility of pressure sores is an ever present danger. If a deep vein thrombosis is diagnosed, passive movements to *both* lower limbs are discontinued because of the possibility of causing a pulmonary embolus.

Movements are recommenced when the anticoagulation therapy is successful.

3. ACTIVE MOVEMENTS

Cervical cord lesions

Gentle, assisted, active movements are given to all innervated muscles from the first day after injury. Progression is made to unassisted active exercises, and the patient is encouraged to move his arms independently and functionally as soon as possible.

Where possible the following movements are taught:

1. Extension of the elbow without triceps
The patient laterally rotates and protracts his shoulder, relaxes biceps and allows gravity to extend the elbow. Independence in this movement should be achieved as soon as possible to prevent shortening of the biceps tendon.

2. To obtain flexion of the shoulder without flexion of the elbow
The patient is encouraged to lift the arm off the bed allowing gravity to keep the elbow extended. Lateral rotation of the shoulder may be necessary initially.

3. To grip without finger movements—wrist extension grip
The grip is obtained by first allowing gravity to flex the wrist when the fingers and thumb fall into extension. The hands or the first finger and thumb are placed over the object to be lifted. Extension of the wrist by extensor carpi radialis places passive tension on the flexors and enables a light object to be held in position. If the object is heavier the pull of gravity can be partially overcome by supinating the forearm.

Although the efficacy of the wrist extension grip can be augmented by allowing some shortening of the finger flexors, not all therapists agree with this approach. Of those who do, some advocate that this shortening should be allowed to develop from the outset but others believe that it should be allowed to occur only when there is no further hope of functional recovery.

Resisted movements

Gentle resisted movements can be gradually introduced as indicated. Strong unilateral exercise for the whole arm involves head movement and is therefore completely avoided until the fracture is healed. All movements must be given with carefully graded resistance avoiding any neck movements.

Neck exercises

Exercises to strengthen the neck extensors may be given in prone lying for 2 weeks before the patient is due to get out of bed. These should be continued during the early weeks of rehabilitation in the wheel chair.

Thoracic cord lesions

Patients with thoracic cord lesions are given frequent resisted arm exercises, either manually or by using a chest expander of suitable strength. All movements are given bilaterally when the pateint is supine, so that resistance is constant and there is no unequal pull on the unstable spine.

FUNCTIONAL ELECTRICAL STIMULATION

Initially functional electrical stimulation is used to improve the condition and bulk of the paralysed muscles. Subsequently electronic implants can be used to activate muscles in functional sequence. Workers in this field hope that eventually paralysed patients will be able to walk independently using a portable computer. It is as yet too early to tell what the influence of this equipment will be on the rehabilitation of the patient with spinal cord injury. Research continues and initial results are encouraging.

6

Pressure — effects and prevention

The direct cause of pressure sores is pressure. It cannot be over-emphasised that pressure sores are caused in bed or in the chair through prolonged *pressure* which prevents adequate circulation to the area.

Contributory factors in patients with spinal cord injury

1. Loss of sensation and voluntary movement

The loss of sensation prevents the patient from receiving warning of long-standing pressure. He is not only unaware of the discomfort normally felt, but due to his immobility he is unable to shift his position to relieve it.

2. Loss of vasomotor control

The impairment of the circulation produces a lowered tissue resistance to pressure. Ischaemia due to local pressure therefore occurs more readily. The vasomotor paralysis is most extreme immediately after injury, and severe sores can be produced very rapidly. Although the vasomotor system is never subsequently normal, some improvement does occur when reflex activity returns to the isolated cord.

Effect of posture

Sores develop mainly over bony prominencies which are exposed to unrelieved pressure in the lying or sitting position. The most vulnerable areas are the sacrum, trochanters, ischial tuberosities, knees, fibulae, malleolii, heels and fifth metatarsals. The occiput and elbows are also at risk in patients with cervical cord lesions. If the patient is placed in a plaster cast sores may also develop over the ribs, spinous processes and anterior and posterior superior iliac spines. Pressure sores also readily occur under splints, plasters, calipers and braces applied over paralysed areas.

Pathology

The pathology may be summarised briefly as follows:

First stage

There is transient circulatory disturbance producing erythema and slight oedema. When pressure is relieved this inflammation disappears within 48 hours.

Second stage

There is permanent damage to the superficial layers of the cutaneous tissues. Vascular stasis occurs, and reddening and congestion of the area does not disappear on digital pressure. The breakdown of skin or the development of blisters is followed by superficial necrosis, and ulcer formation.

Third stage

There is penetrating and frequently extensive necrosis with destruction of subcutaneous tissue, fascia, muscles and bone. If the infection extends to the bone, periostitis and osteomyelitis will develop, which may result in the destruction of joints and the formation of ectopic bone. If unchecked these major lesions may lead to general septicaemia and death.

Development of bursae

A bursa can develop, frequently over the ischial tuberosity, due to prolonged sitting. The surrounding tissues are rapidly involved if infection occurs, and a very small skin opening may be the only visible sign of a deep cavity reaching down to the infected bursa, and usually to bone.

The prevention of pressure sores

'Where there is no pressure, there will be no sore.'

Prevention, therefore, depends primarily upon the frequent relief of pressure in conjunction with the correct positioning of the patient (see Ch. 5).

Turning the patient

Patients are turned every 2 hours, day and night, using the supine and side lying positions.

Besides preventing the effects of prolonged pressure regular turning also aids renal function by preventing stagnation in the urinary tract. The most susceptible areas, that is, where bony points are close to the skin, must be kept free of any pressure by adjusting the pillows accordingly. At each turn all such areas are inspected, the skin is checked and all wrinkles and debris removed from the bed linen. Any evidence of local pressure, however minor, is an urgent warning. Redness, which does not fade on pressure, septic spots, bruising, swelling, induration or grazing indicate an impending pressure sore. All pressure must be relieved from any area thus affected until it is healed. For example if the sacrum shows signs of redness the left and right lateral positions only should be used until the mark has completely disappeared.

At the National Spinal Injuries Centre the Egerton-Stoke Mandeville Electrical Turning and Tilting Bed is currently used to facilitate the 2-hourly turning of patients. This bed is divided longitudinally into three sections. On pressing a button two of these sections elevate to 70°. The remaining third can be slightly raised to maintain the patient in position. The head and foot of the bed will tilt down to 15°. The Guttmann head traction unit is applied when skull traction is required. This unit enables constant cervical traction to be maintained when turning the patient. A face piece supports the head in the lateral position. The senior nurse organises each turn and ensures that correct spinal alignment is maintained whilst the patient is moved.

If the Egerton bed is not available, the patient can be positioned on a bed with sorbo-rubber packs. The space between the packs is altered to suit the position and stature of the patient so that the bony prominences are free from pressure. The prone position is particularly useful for the nonacute lesion if the sores are on the sacrum, trochanters or ischii, or on all three sites. In this position care must be taken to ensure that the toes, knees, iliac crests and genital areas are clear of pressure (Fig. 6.1). Support to the back is given by sandbags when in the side lying position.

If sorbo packs are not available pillow packs can be used. These are made by tying five or six pillows tightly together.

Body support systems are constantly being developed to facilitate the healing of pressure sores. A current example is the low air loss bed system in which the pressure in each of several sections is controlled individually according to the patient's requirements.

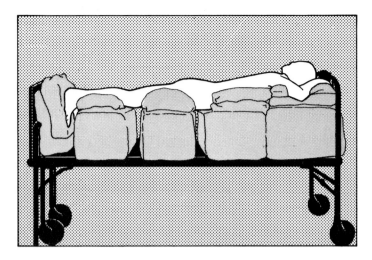

Fig. 6.1 Prone position of patient on a pack bed.

Care of the skin

The emphasis is on cleanliness and dryness.

Intact skin is kept clean by the normal use of soap and water. No local applications of methyl alcohol, etc., are used. Dead epithelium tends to collect through disuse on the soles of the feet and palms of the hands. It can be prevented and removed by thoroughly washing and towelling these areas and then rubbing in lanolin.

PRESSURE CONSCIOUSNESS: RE-EDUCATION IN SELFCARE OF THE DESENSITISED AREAS

Whilst the patient is in bed the prevention of pressure sores is the responsibility of the medical team. As soon as he is mobile this responsibility must be transferred to the patient if he is to remain free from pressure sores in the future.

Lifting

To allow adequate circulation to be maintained in the areas of maximum pressure, relief of pressure at regular intervals is essential. In the sitting position maximum weight is taken on the ischial tuberosities. Therefore as soon as the patient sits in the wheelchair the therapist must teach him to 'lift' the weight off his buttocks. The simplest lift is achieved by pushing down on the armrests, straightening the elbows and *depressing the shoulders*. Lifting and repositioning should be done slowly and carefully. Patients with cervical lesions may be able to lift only one side at a time, and those without triceps need to hyperextend the elbows (Fig. 6.2).

The ability to lift primarily depends upon the level of the lesion, although other factors such as overweight or associated fractures of the arms will obviously influence it.

Various methods of lifting for patients with lesions at different levels are shown in Figure 6.2. The position of the hands and trunk and the use of the head will vary considerably in patients with cervical lesions.

All patients are instructed to 'lift' for at least 10 seconds once every 10 minutes, including meal times and when out socially, e.g. visits to the cinema. This will gradually become second nature and the patient will lift automatically. Until that time he will need to be frequently reminded and encouraged. If required various pressure gauges with alarm systems are available to assist the patient to remember to lift.

Depending on the level of the lesion the patient may be able to lift at the first session of instruction or require weeks of training, or it may never be within the physical capabilities of the patient. Those unable to lift themselves must be lifted by the staff at least every half-hour.

Lifting a patient to relieve pressure

1. Stand in step standing behind the wheelchair with the patient sitting well back in the seat.
2. Flex the patient's trunk and cross his forearms over his lower ribs.
3. Grasp the patient's forearms (Fig. 6.3a).
4. Lift the patient, and at the same time grip with the forearms around the lower ribcage and extend the hips.
5. Take the patient's weight on the thigh of the forward leg (Fig. 6.3b).
6. Lower gently after 30 seconds.

Turning at night

The patient must also become responsible for the prevention of pressure occurring during the night. He must learn to turn himself in bed every 3 hours, to reposition the pillows between the legs and ensure as far as possible that he is not lying on any creases in the bed linen.

Inspection of the skin

Care of the desensitised and paralysed areas of the body must form an integral part of the patient's daily life. He must learn to inspect his skin night and morning for pressure marks, abrasions and septic

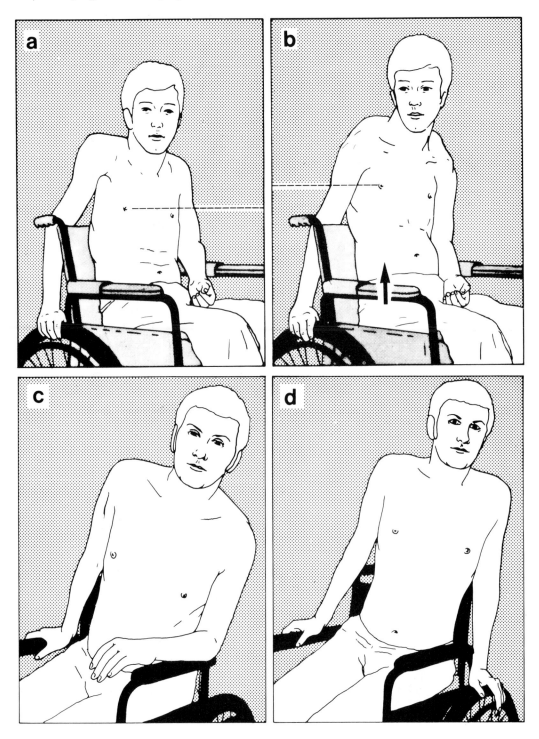

Fig. 6.2 Lifting in the wheelchair. (a & b) Patient with a complete lesion below C_5. (c) Patient with a complete lesion below C_6 without triceps. (d) Patient with a complete lesion below C_7 with wrist control only.

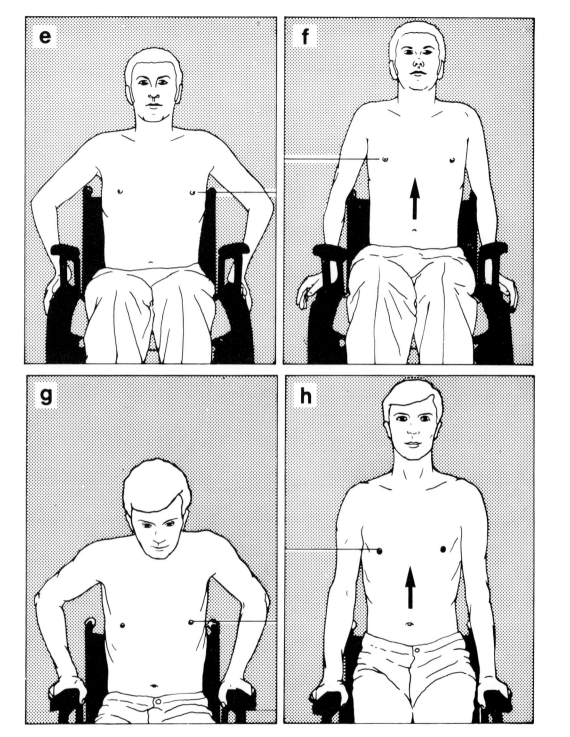

Fig. 6.2 (contd) (e & f) Patient with a complete lesion below C_7 with wrist control only. (g & h) Patient with a complete lesion below T_5.

spots. Special attention is given to the most vulnerable areas, that is, the sacral, ischial and trochanteric areas, plus the knees, malleolii and toes. A mirror is used to inspect any areas the patient cannot view directly. Those patients who are unable to inspect their own skin must be responsible to ask for this to be done.

Patients able to lift themselves usually sit on a 4-inch (10 cm) sorbo cushion in the wheelchair. As the resilience of these cushions rapidly diminishes due to hard wear, the patient should examine his cushion regularly and have it replaced when necessary. Those patients unable to lift themselves will need a special cushion, such as a foam or gel emulsion cushion, or the roho dry floatation cushion.

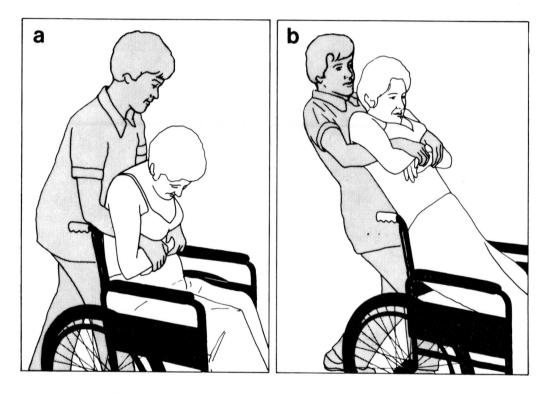

Fig. 6.3 Lifting a patient to relieve pressure.

The paralysed limbs

Great care must be taken in lifting the limbs whenever the patient transfers. A bruise sustained by knocking the malleolus against the foot plate, for example, can become a deep sore and take weeks and even months to heal. Bruises devitalize the overlying skin and should be treated as pressure marks. As the vasomotor system does not allow adjustments of the circulation, care must be taken also to ensure that the desensitised areas are protected from excessive heat or cold.

Do's and dont's

The patient is taught the following list of simple 'do's and don'ts' when he first gets out of bed:

Do lift in the chair every 10 minutes.

Do lift the paralysed limbs when transferring.

Do use a mirror for detection of marks, abrasions, blisters, redness on buttocks, back of legs and malleoli.

Do watch for marks on the penis from the condom.

Do protect the limbs against excessive cold.

Do have the bath water ready and not too hot.

Don't open the hot tap when having a bath in case hot water drips on the toes.

Don't have a hot water bottle in bed.

Don't expose the body to strong sunlight; tetraplegic patients must wear a hat.

Don't knock the limbs against any hard object.

Don't carry hot drinks on the lap.

Don't rest the paralysed limbs on hot water pipes or radiators.

Don't sit too close to the fire.

Don't leave the legs, particularly the feet, unprotected against car heaters.

7

Initial physical re-education

As soon as the spine has consolidated and the general condition permits, the patient is allowed to sit up in bed prior to sitting in a wheelchair. A reinforced plastazote, or plastic support, may be worn for 2 or 3 weeks to prevent acute flexion until the spinal musculature becomes stronger. An anterior shell, held in position with three webbing and velcro straps, is used for patients with thoracic lesions. Those with cervical lesions use an anterior collar, which holds the neck in the anatomical position (Fig. 7.1).

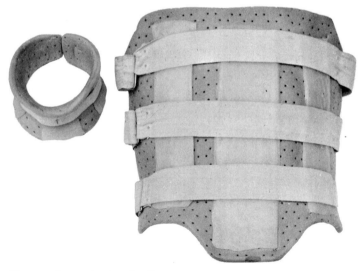

Fig. 7.1 'Breastplate' and collar.

Electrically operated beds are available which move into a full sitting position in which the patient's hips and knees are flexed and his feet are down. The use of this type of bed obviates the need to sit in long sitting and risk putting any stretch on the dura mater. The bed, which can be operated by the patient or an attendant is also useful in controlling postural hypotension.

Programme for patient's activities

As soon as the patient is out of bed the physiotherapist, occupational therapist and ward sister liaise to work out a programme of increasing activity for each patient according to his individual needs.

Initially the patient will attend the physiotherapy and occupational therapy departments for only a short period, approximately $\frac{1}{2}$–1 hour in each department. Gradually, as the patient is able to stay up for longer periods the programme is increased. By the end of 7–10 days the paraplegic patient will be achieving a full day's programme working from 0900 to 1700. Most tetraplegic patients will take at least 3 weeks to achieve this. These assessments of time will depend, as always, on the patient's age, general state of health and previous medical history. Each patient receives a written timetable, and a copy is given to the ward sister.

AIMS OF TREATMENT

The ultimate aim of rehabilitation is to achieve the highest degree of fitness, independence, balance and control which the patient's lesion permits. This is to be achieved by re-education and the fullest possible use of each muscle over which the patient has voluntary control. The immediate aims of treatment therefore are:

1. Readjustment of the vasomotor control.
2. Re-education of postural sensibility.
3. The re-education and hyperdevelopment of the normal parts of the body to compensate for the paralysed muscles. The fulfillment of these aims is the foundation for restoring independence (Figs 7.2 & 7.3).
4. The education of the patient in self-care of the desensitised areas (see Ch. 6).

VASOMOTOR DISTURBANCE

Postural hypotension is particularly common in patients with cervical or high thoracic lesions. This is due primarily to loss of vasomotor control in the splanchnic area. The blood vessels in the viscera are unable to constrict when the body is raised from the horizontal to the vertical position. The vasomotor control which is lost cannot be regained, but the patient can overcome the disturbance by developing other vascular reflexes which are still intact.

The reflexes are trained in a variety of ways, by means of deep breathing exercises, tilting exercises in bed, frequent changes of

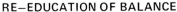

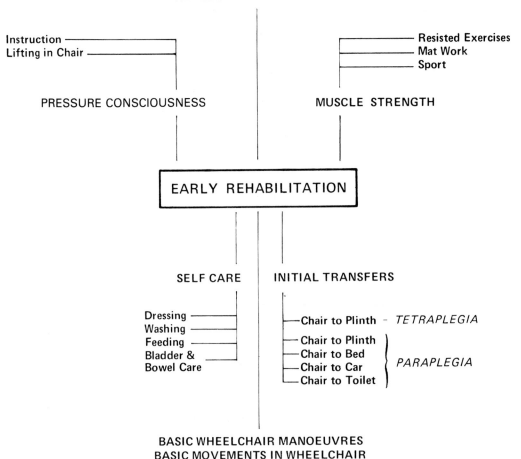

Fig. 7.2 Early physical rehabilitation.

position and graduated balance exercises in the sitting and standing positions.

Before sitting out in the wheelchair the patient is tilted in the bed. Gradual progression is made from the initial 30° until the patient can sit at 90° without feeling faint. Deep breathing exercises are given in each position. The time in the tilted position is lengthened gradually from ½–3 hours over approximately a week. The skin over the ischii and coccyx is not accustomed to weight-bearing. Constant inspection is necessary as a pressure sore can easily develop.

Whilst sitting the paraplegic patient should practise lifting his body weight on his hands. He can either push down on the bed or use wooden lifting blocks if available. This exercise helps to establish the vascular reflexes, increases the strength of latissimus dorsi, and relieves pressure on the buttocks.

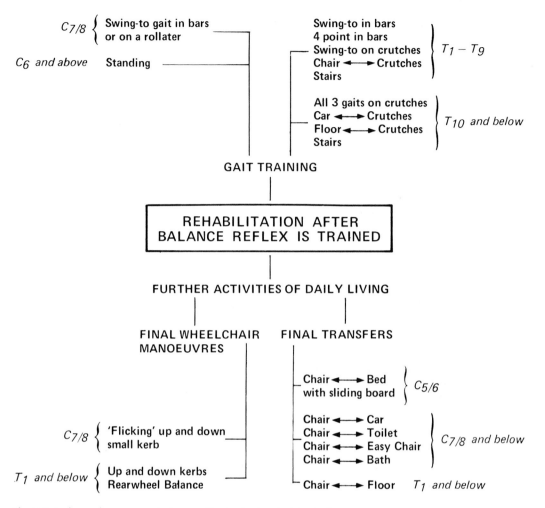

Fig. 7.3 Independence expected according to the level of the lesion.

When vasomotor control is established in the bed, training is commenced in the wheelchair, initially for a few moments at a time. The process of gradually and regularly extending the time is repeated.

Active rehabilitation in the various departments commences when the patient can tolerate 3 hours in the wheelchair. At first the patient will need to be pushed to the departments. As he has not experienced motion of any kind for several weeks, even relatively slow speeds will seem alarmingly fast. As soon as possible the patient should push himself and be responsible for keeping his own appointments.

Fainting

As fainting can occur it is advisable not to leave the patient alone during the early days of vasomotor training in the wheelchair.

If the patient complains of feeling faint or dizzy, has blurred vision or appears white and sweaty the legs must be elevated and the chair tipped on to its rear wheels immediately. Deep breathing is encouraged by giving pressure during expiration over the lower ribs and upper abdomen. Should loss of consciousness occur with no signs of recovery within a minute, the patient should be placed flat.

The vasomotor problem must be explained to the patient. Instructions should be given on how to aid the circulation when feeling faint by brisk movements of the arms and deep breathing.

Encouragement is essential, as once a patient has fainted, fear of a recurrence may inhibit his activity.

POSTURAL SENSIBILITY

The patient with a complete spinal cord lesion has lost not only sensibility to touch, pain and temperature and motor power of the trunk and limbs, but also his postural or kinesthetic sense, below the level of the lesion.

> Kinesthesia is the perception of the position and movement of one's body parts in space. It also includes perception of the internal and external tensions and forces tending to move or stabilise a joint.
>
> Rasch & Burke, 1971

In complete lesions above T_{12} where postural sensibility in the hip joints is abolished, the patient has difficulty in keeping his balance in the unsupported upright position. The development of a new postural sense is a major objective in the rehabilitation of these patients. It is the foundation for all daily living activities.

Postural control is achieved largely through those muscles which have a high innervation and low distal attachment. These muscles form a bridge between the normal parts of the body, including of course the brain, and the paralysed areas. The most important of these muscles is latissimus dorsi. It has a high segmental supply $(C_{6,7,8})$ and an extensive attachment to the spine and pelvis. Therefore in all lesions below C_7 it bridges the paralysed and nonparalysed parts of the body and allows patients with high thoracic and low cervical cord lesions to regain a high degree of balance and control.

> Proprioceptive impulses arising from any movement of the pelvis are transmitted centrally along the afferent nerve fibres of these normally innervated muscles and thus reconnect the insensitive part of the body with the cerebral and cerebellar centres promoting appropriate efferent postural responses to the paralysed area. . . . Eventually a new pattern of postural sensibility develops along the nerve supply of the trunk muscles.
>
> Guttmann, 1973

Latissimus dorsi is important both in the restoration of the paraplegic's upright position and in his future gait training. The function
of this muscle is greatly assisted by other trunk and shoulder girdle
muscles, particularly trapezius because of its dorsal attachment as
low as T_{12} and the abdominal muscles with their insertion on the
pelvis.

The patient develops his new postural sense primarily by visual
control. He performs exercises sitting in front of a mirror where he
can see the position of his body and limbs. This visual-motor
feedback helps him gradually to develop more acute sensory im-
pressions, i.e. interpreting the muscle stretch sensations of the
latissimus dorsi and other trunk muscles, and a new sensorial pattern
becomes established.

He will then perform movements not only without the aid of a
mirror but without conscious effort for functional activities.

Balance exercises in the sitting position

These exercises are primarily carried out sitting on the plinth, in front
of the mirror though some patients may need to begin their exercises
sitting in the wheelchair (see p. 72).

Position of the patient

1. The patient sits well back on a low plinth in front of a long mirror.
A pillow is placed under the buttocks to guard against excessive
pressure.

2. The thighs and feet are well supported so that a right angle is
formed at the hips, knees and ankles.

Role of the therapist

1. The therapist stands behind the patient so that she can watch
his movements in the mirror and have control should he lose balance.

2. Her hands initially support the patient either over the shoulders
or round the thorax. Her hands should be visible to the patient.
Should she put them where he cannot feel, he is unaware of the
support and confidence is lost.

3. Assurance is given that the therapist will not move away. The
fear of falling, especially backwards, is very marked. The therapist
should never leave her position unless the patient has some form of
support, as he can easily overbalance and fall off the plinth. The
position is obviously more dangerous for those with severe spasticity.

4. The therapist can to a large extent control the speed of the
patient's activity by her voice and her general handling of the

situation. Her voice should be quiet and confident and, most important of all, unhurried since all exercises involving balance must be performed *slowly*.

5. She should give constant direction and encouragement.

6. When the patient overbalances, the therapist should allow a gross movement to occur before restraining him, otherwise the patient may not be aware of the movement that has taken place.

Progression of exercises

1. Self-supported sitting

Watching himself in the mirror the patient learns to support himself in as upright a position as possible with his hands first on the plinth at his sides, then on his knees. If the lesion is high and the arms are short in relation to the trunk, it may help to have a pillow at each side of the patient to support the hands. Time and trouble should be taken to teach the patient to hold the correct sitting position before commencing exercises involving motion.

2. Single arm exercises

Always watching himself closely in the mirror the patient raises one arm first sideways, then forwards and lastly upwards whilst supporting himself with the other hand on his knee. A small degree of movement of the head and trunk to the side of the supporting hand will be necessary to compensate for the weight of the moving arm. Single arm exercises are not found to be helpful for patients with lesions at C_6 or above, since without triceps the supporting arm is ineffective.

3. Bilateral arm exercises

Larger compensatory movements of the head and trunk will be necessary when moving both arms in the unsupported sitting position. The patient first tries to hold the arms in the bend position then progresses to raising both arms sideways, forwards, upwards (Fig. 7.4).

The sideways stretch position presents little difficulty since the centre of gravity is barely altered.

In the forwards stretch position the patient must lean his head and body backwards to counteract the line of gravity which would otherwise fall in front of the hip joints.

The upward stretch position is particularly difficult for patients with high lesions, since the centre of gravity is raised and the patient has no abdominal muscles to help him to maintain his equilibrium.

4. Bilateral arm exercises without the mirror

When the patient has mastered the basic positions and exercises, bilateral exercises are performed without the mirror and with the eyes closed.

5. Other exercises

Balance can be further improved by for example asymmetrical work, altering the rate of movement, resisted trunk exercises, stabilisations and ball throwing.

Duration and frequency of treatment

These exercises are physically and mentally exhausting. Treatment is given daily for only 5–10 minutes initially, progressing to half-an-hour. Frequent rests should be given during treatment by allowing the patient to lean back against the therapist for a few moments. Tetraplegic patients need to rest the head to allow the neck extensors to relax. Balance training requires constant practice and it is valuable to treat patients with thoracic lesions twice daily.

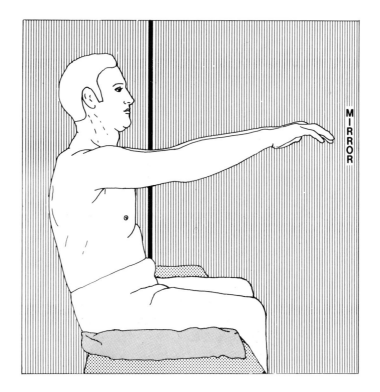

Fig. 7.4 Balance position of a patient with a complete lesion below T_6.

Patients with low thoracic lesions should be trained in 1–2 weeks. Those with high thoracic lesions may take up to 6 weeks and those with cervical lesions will probably need 3–8 weeks or longer.

These estimates of time are generalisations only, dependent as always upon the usual limits imposed by age, stature and previous medical history.

Balance in the wheelchair

Balance exercises are commenced in the wheelchair for the following reasons:

1. Poor posture when sitting on the plinth

This occurs:

a. with high cervical lesions, C_5 or above, when the head pokes forward and the patient is unable to extend the neck.

b. with some thoracic lesions when the trunk is flexed, due to weak extensor muscles. It may be necessary for such patients to concentrate on back extension exercises for a week, balancing only in the wheelchair. When the general muscle tone has improved the patient can return to balance exercises on the plinth.

2. General debility

The patient may not be fit to be moved in and out of the chair.

3. Recently healed sores

The scar tissue may be delicate. Movement in and out of the wheelchair may constitute a potential danger until the scar tissue becomes stronger.

Exercises in the wheelchair are carried out in front of the mirror as described above, first leaning against the back of the chair and progressing to sitting away from the back rest. As soon as possible balance on the plinth should be commenced or resumed.

Posture

Although the aim is to achieve as upright a position as possible, this will vary according to the level of the lesion. The *low thoracic lesion* (with abdominal muscles) should have a straight back.

The *upper thoracic lesion* (without abdominal muscles) has a typical posture with increased kyphosis and lordosis.

The *low cervical lesion* usually has a good, straight posture providing trapezius is strong and the patient has not been allowed to sit on his sacrum for several weeks or months, producing a long kyphosis.

The *high cervical lesion* as a rule has a poor posture with poking head and flexed spine.

Sport

Archery and table tennis are useful activites in training postural control.

MUSCLE RE-EDUCATION

To establish a satisfactory compensatory mechanism to cope with the paralysed limbs all innervated muscles need to be as strong as possible. For patients with complete lesions it is particularly important where possible to hypertrophy the following:

1. latissimus dorsi
2. shoulder and shoulder girdle muscles, particularly adductors
3. arm muscles
4. abdominal muscles.

The choice of technique for strengthening these muscles belongs to the individual therapist. The choice will depend upon her past experience and training, personal preference and possibly the staff/patient ratio.

Methods currently used include:

1. manual resistance, including proprioceptive neuromuscular facilitation (PNF) techniques
2. spring and sling suspension therapy
3. weights and pulleys
4. sport.

Where the staff/patient ratio is high, PNF is particularly useful for:

1. patients with incomplete lesions with very little spasticity
2. strengthening the trunk muscles
3. strengthening the arms of patients with cervical lesions.

In the absence of more sophisticated systems bilateral strengthening exercises for latissimus dorsi and the pectoral muscles can be given to paraplegic patients by a simple system of weights and pulleys (Fig. 7.5). With the pulley handles at shoulder level, the patient pulls down to the chair wheels keeping the elbows straight. If

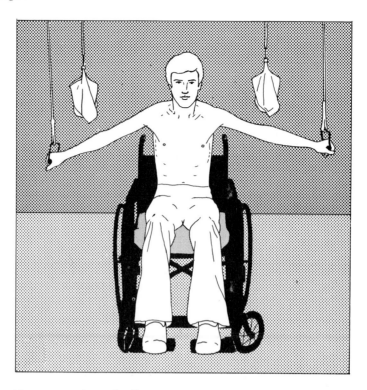

Fig. 7.5 Weights and pulleys used to strengthen latissimus dorsi.

the elbows are allowed to flex, the exercise becomes one to strengthen triceps and not latissimus dorsi as desired.

Body weight is useful as resistance in free exercises such as pressups and lifting up on blocks.

Progression

In all exercise programmes progression must be carefully graded both for strength and endurance and for the effect on cardio-respiratory function. It is often helpful for the patient to watch himself in a mirror when performing his exercises to get some visuospatial feedback.

Biofeedback can be useful in muscle re-education. It assists the patient to strive for maximum effort and enables him to measure his achievement.

8

Self-care

Close co-operation between the occupational therapist and physio-therapist is essential in planning the patient's rehabilitation pro-gramme. The work of the two disciplines complement one another and in many areas overlap.

All but those with the highest lesions must learn to dress, and in addition tetraplegic patients must learn to eat and drink, brush the hair, clean the teeth, wash and shave. For all practical purposes patients without finger movement can be divided into three groups: those with lesions at C_4, C_5 and C_6.

Patients with lesions at C_4

These patients are without any muscle power in the upper limbs. By means of appropriate mouth sticks, with a dental bite (Fig. 8.1), they can learn to turn the pages of a small paper or magazine, type, paint and play board games where the pieces have been suitably adapted (see Ch. 13 The Ultra-High Lesion).

Patients with lesions at C_5

These patients have good functioning deltoids and biceps but no muscle control at the wrist. A light cock-up splint is used to stabilise the wrist joint. This contains a slot in the palmar surface to hold simple gadgets such as a spoon, fork or typing stick (Fig. 8.1a). With practice most patients at this level learn to eat, type, move papers using a stick with a rubber cap and play games such as draughts, chess, dominoes with specially adapted pieces.

Patients with lesions at C_6

These patients have an active extensor carpi radialis and are able to pick up objects by using the wrist extension grip. Patients with lesions

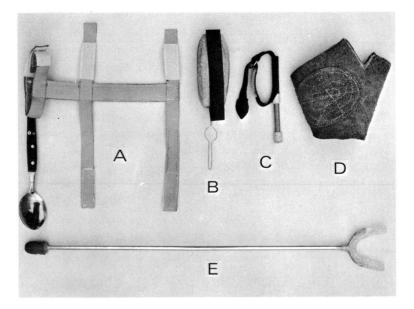

Fig. 8.1 (A) Wrist splint with spoon for patient with a complete lesion below C_5. (B) Button hook. (C) Typing stock in strap used by patient with a complete lesion below C_6. (D) Pushing glove. (E) Mouth stick.

at C_7 without finger movement can be included in this group, although the active elbow extension and wrist flexion gives greater dexterity in all activities.

As a weak grip can be sustained, these patients can achieve a measure of independence in the wheelchair.

The grip is practised and the patient taught to pick up everyday objects of different sizes, to manipulate paper and to turn the pages of books and magazines. A small leather strap with a slot in the palmar surface is used to hold various implements for daily living. (Fig. 8.1C) The strap is both light and unobtrusive and the patient can put it on unaided. After the initial period of training, most of these patients become so skilful in using their hands that gadgets are rendered unnecessary.

The flexor hinge splint, which utilises extensor carpi radialis to produce a pincer grip, can be a useful asset to some patients, especially those who return to work. Modular kits are available which enable the splint to be fitted and in use within a few days.

SELF-CARE FOR PATIENTS WITH LESIONS AT C_6

Feeding

Patients start to eat by using the strap to hold the fork or spoon and extending and relaxing the wrist. After some practice the strap is usually discarded and the fork held by balancing it over the thumb and against the palm of the hand or over the little finger. A plate guard may be helpful initially.

Drinking

A cup or mug with a large handle is held by hooking the thumb through the handle and extending the wrist. A glass without a handle can be lifted by sliding the fingers and thumb around the glass with the wrist extensor relaxed and then extending the wrist to produce the necessary grip.

As the hands are insensitive and the movements slow and clumsy, insulated mugs are preferred whilst training. Standard cups are used later by most dexterous patients.

Cleaning the teeth

The toothbrush is used in the strap or laced between the fingers. To unscrew the cap from the toothpaste tube, the cap can be held by the teeth, whilst both hands rotate the tube. The teeth can also be used to squeeze out the paste.

Brushing the hair

Most patients find a shampoo brush with a wide handle easy to use.

Shaving

To enable the patient to shave unaided a soft leather jacket can be sewn around the electric shaver and a strap attached to fit over the dorsum of the hand. Many patients learn to use the razor without the jacket. The patient manoeuvres the razor into position between the fingers and palm of the right hand, with the head of the razor projecting between the thumb and first finger. He then places his left hand round the other to strengthen the grip. By pressing the two hands together the grip is maintained.

Dressing

Dressing training is commenced as soon as the spine is stable.

Upper-extremity dressing refers to the ability to put on and remove clothing over the upper limbs.

Lower-extremity dressing refers to the ability to put on and remove clothing over the lower limbs.

Total dressing refers to the ability to achieve both the foregoing.

Although most paraplegic patients will finally achieve total dressing both in bed and in the wheelchair, they are initially taught to dress in bed. Tetraplegic patients need to gain some sitting balance before attempting to dress, and it is usual to begin with upper-extremity dressing in the wheelchair. Each patient, having learnt the basic methods, will find an individual way which best suits his requirements and daily schedule.

Caution *Training is delayed where there is: (a) instability of the spine at the site of the injury, (b) delicate scar tissue which might easily break down during rolling or through friction.*

Clothing

All clothing should be loose-fitting. The trousers need to be at least a size larger than normally worn to accommodate the urinal and avoid trauma due to friction. Zips in a side seam of the trouser leg are also a help if wearing a urinal or calipers. A wrap-over skirt and rubber pants with a front fastening may be helpful for female patients who find difficulty in removing clothing for toilet purposes.

Shoes a half to one size larger than those worn prior to the paralysis are usually required to avoid pressure sores and accommodate for any oedema or spasticity. They should have smooth inside seams, must remain in position when the legs are lifted and should be selected according to the patient's needs.

For tetraplegic patients zips or velcro fastenings are the most easily managed. Since the thumb is used as a hook on many occasions, loops or split rings on the zipper pulls may be helpful. Brassieres should have stretch straps and should not be boned, because of the danger of pressure marks.

Loose woollen socks are easier to put on initially. Progression can be made to nylon socks later if desired.

Clip-on ties may be useful for some patients with cervical lesions.

Level of lesion in relation to dressing

Total dressing should be achieved by patients with lesions as high as C_7, that is, patients with active flexion and extension of elbows and wrists.

Total dressing may be achieved by patients with lesions at C_6 both with or without triceps, but lower-extremity dressing for these patients, though useful in emergency, is usually so costly in time that it is not practical. Upper-extremity dressing should be achieved by patients with lesions at C_{5-6} except for the following activities:

to put on a brassiere

to tuck the shirt tails into the trouser band
to fasten buttons on cuffs and shirt fronts.

Patients without figer movement cannot usually manage to put on the condom urinal.

As always these objectives are only possible within the limits imposed by the previous medical history, the age and the physical proportions of the patient.

DRESSING TECHNIQUES

In most movements two actions are involved:
1. to move the garment
2. to move the body, that is, to wriggle into or out of the garment.

Balance

Those tetraplegic patients who can lift in the chair during dressing should put the stronger hand towards the back of the armrest, with the forearm braced against the backrest support and the weaker hand towards the front of the armrest. This arrangement gives more stability anteroposteriorly and allows wriggling movements forwards and backwards as well as from side to side.

Patients who find difficulty in maintaining balance whilst using both arms are more stable if the buttocks are brought a few inches forwards in the chair.

Spasticity

A certain degree of spasticity may be an advantage in flexing and extending the lower limbs. Uncontrollable muscle spasm in the lower limbs may render independent dressing impossible. Sitting cross-legged for 15–20 minutes may help reduce severe spasticity before attempting to dress.

As it is easier to achieve, the tetraplegic patient is taught to undress first. However, for clarity in the following section the method for putting the garment on is described first. This procedure is usually reversed when taking it off.

Dressing in the wheelchair

Upper-extremity dressing in a wheelchair

As upper-extremity dressing provides no problem for low lesions, i.e. those with abdominals, reference in this section is to patients with cervical and high thoracic lesions.

Putting on a garment of soft material with or without a front fastening

This method can be used for blouses, vests, sweaters, skirts and dresses that open down the front. If it is found easier and the garment is large enough, the buttons can be left fastened. Many tetraplegic patients without a grip can learn to fasten buttons by using a button hook (Fig. 8.1B).

1. Position the garment on the thighs, with the neckline towards the knees.

2. Put both arms under the back of the garment and through the armholes.

3. Push the garment past the elbows.

4. Using the wrist extension grip, hook the thumbs under the garment and gather the material up from the neck to hem.

5. Using adduction and lateral rotation of the shoulders and flexion of the elbows and neck, pass the garment over the head.

6. Relax the shoulders and wrists and remove the hands from the back of the garment. Most of the material will be gathered up at the back of the neck and under the arms.

7. There are several ways in which the garment can be worked down into place:

   a. Shrug the shoulders and/or elevate and laterally rotate the shoulders with the elbows extended to get the material down across the shoulders.

   b. Hook the wrists into the sleeves and pull the material free at the axilla.

   c. Using two hands pull down on each side of the front.

   d. Hook one hand in the material at the neck, lean on the opposite forearm on the armrest and pull the garment down.

Taking the garment off

1. Hook the thumb in the back of the neckline, extend the wrist and pull the garment over the head turning the head towards the side of the raised arm. Maintain balance by either:

   a. leaning on the opposite forearm or

   b. pushing the thigh with the extended arm.

2. Hook the thumb in the opposite armhole and push the sleeve down the arm. Pull the arm out of the garment.

Putting on a jacket

1. Put the weaker arm in the armhole and push the sleeve up the arm.

2. Maintain balance by leaning on and over the forearm resting on the armrest.

3. Put the other arm in the armhole behind the back.

4. Elevate the arms and shrug the shoulders to get the jacket over the shoulders.

Removing a jacket

Reverse the above procedure.

Putting on a brassiere with fastening at the back

1. Powder under the breasts and round the chest wall, especially if subject to sweating attacks.

2. Place bra on the knees, inside out and upside down, i.e. with the lower edge of the bra towards the knees.

3. Balance on the weaker elbow. Hold the middle of the bra with the strong hand, take behind the back and bring the fastening to the front.

4. Fasten the hooks or velcro at the front. It may help to lift slightly on the forearms.

5. Wriggle the bra round to the back. Powder again if necessary.

6. With the thumbs in the strap pull up over breasts.

7. Place one arm at a time in the appropriate shoulder strap. Hook the thumb under the bra strap, lean to the opposite side and put the strap over the shoulder. Repeat for the other arm.

8. Look in the mirror to see that the bra is not wrinkled.

Note Adjust the length of the straps when the bra is off.

Taking off the brassiere

1. Hook the thumb under the opposite strap, and push down whilst elevating the shoulder.

2. Pull the arm out of the strap.

3. Repeat on the other side.

4. Push the bra down and turn it round to bring the fastening to the front.

5. Undo the fastening.

Lower-extremity dressing in the wheelchair

When dressing the lower extremity the socks should be put on before the trousers to avoid catching the toes and causing trauma.

Putting on and removing socks and shoes

Whether in the chair or on the bed maximum control is achieved when putting on and taking off socks and shoes by crossing one ankle over the opposite knee. The tetraplegic patient uses the wrist extension grip and the palm of the hands in a patting movement to pull on the socks.

Putting on trousers

1. Lift the right leg with the right wrist behind the knee and the forearm on the armrest. Put the trouser leg over the foot. Repeat with the left leg.
  Or, cross the right ankle over left knee, put the trousers over the foot and pull up to knee height. Replace the right foot on the footplate. Repeat with the left leg.
2. Pull the trousers well up over the knees and under the thighs, lean on the left forearm and lift the right knee with the left wrist to pull the trousers up the thigh.
3. Hook the right fingers or thumb inside the back of the waistband, lean over to the left and lift on the left hand and forearm. Repeat from side to side. At each lift wriggle forwards and backwards whilst the buttocks are in the air.

Alternative methods to pull the trousers over the buttocks for paraplegic patients

1. Lean forwards on the forearms on the armrests, depressing the shoulders and lifting the buttocks, and pull the trousers up.
2. Lean well back taking the weight on the top of the backrest, wriggle the buttocks forwards and at the same time pull up the trousers.

Dressing on the bed

Upper-extremity dressing on the bed

This presents no real problems for paraplegic patients. Tetraplegic patients have more stability for upper-extremity dressing in the wheelchair and rarely do it on the bed.

Lower-extremity dressing on the bed

Putting on trousers

1. Put the trouser legs over the feet as for the socks.
2. Flex the knee with the hand, wrist or forearm and pull the trousers up over the thighs. Lean on the elbows if necessary.
3. Repeat for the other leg.

4. Lean to the right on the right elbow, pull the trousers over the left buttock.

5. Lean to the left and pull the trousers over the right buttock. Repeat this as often as necessary.

A monkey pole may be necessary for patients with high thoracic lesions to lift on to the side at the commencement of training.

Remove the trousers by reversing the procedure

Alternative method for tetraplegic patients

1. Sit up, hook the right hand under the right knee and pull the knee into flexion.

2. Put the trousers over the right foot.

3. Repeat for the left foot. It may help to have both legs slightly flexed and laterally rotated at the hips.

4. Work the trousers up the legs by alternately flexing the knees and using a patting sliding motion with the palms of the hands.

5. Lie down and pull the right knee onto the chest.

6. Stay supine and hold the right knee with the left forearm or roll into left side lying. Throw the right arm behind the back, hook the thumb in the waistband or belt loops, or the hand in the trouser pocket, and pull the trousers over the right buttock.

7. Repeat for the other side. These steps may need to be repeated several times until the trousers are in place over the hips.

8. Fasten the trouser placket by hooking the thumb in a loop on the zipper pull.

If the patient cannot cross one ankle over the other, the trousers, socks and shoes have to be put over the feet in long sitting. This is more difficult since the heels are resting on the bed.

Writing

There are several gadgets used to hold a pen or pencil. Most tetraplegic patients give up the gadgets in time and either lace the pen through their fingers or hold it in one hand, putting the other hand on top to reinforce the grip.

Typing

Most patients type with a small, rubber-tipped wooden stick set in a balsa wood handle with a strap over the dorsum of the hand (Fig. 8.1C). The forearms are held in mid-position and where possible both hands are used. The patient with a C_4 lesion who has the mental ability to master the technique may prefer to use a possum typewriter to typing with a mouth stick. The possum typewriter control system is mouth-operated by gentle suction and/or pressure down a tube.

Computers and word processors can be used for both work and leisure activities as they can be manipulated with a stick held either in a strap on the hand or in the mouth.

Using the telephone

The post office will adapt a telephone to allow the patient with an ultra-high lesion to make independent calls. If these adaptations are not available the receiver can be mounted on a retort stand and a simple wooden bar with a firm handle placed across the receiver rest. A mouth stick can be used to dial and to remove and replace the wooden bar.

Housework

Both low tetraplegic and paraplegic female patients prepare for their return to housekeeping in the occupational therapy department kitchen and in the ward. They dust, cook, wash up, make their own beds and do their own laundry. They have the opportunity to discuss ways and means to overcome individual problems in the home and in this way gain the necessary confidence to return to their family responsibility.

Electronic equipment, such as that produced by possum, will be needed by the patient with an ultra-high lesion, if he is to have any control over his home environment.

Bladder, bowel and skin care

The care of the bladder and bowels is dealt with in Chapter 3 and re-education in self-care of the desensitised areas in Chapter 6.

9

Mat work

Activities on the mat will include:

1. Mobilisation and strengthening of the trunk and limbs.
2. Preliminary training for functional activities.

MOBILISATION AND STRENGTHENING OF THE TRUNK AND LIMBS

Some degree of stiffness in the trunk will result from the weeks of immobility in bed. In addition there will be some shortening of the hamstring muscles. If the activities of daily living are to be mastered, good mobility is essential.

Therefore mobilisation of the trunk in all directions and stretching of any tight muscle groups is an essential part of early rehabilitation. Active assisted, active and resisted work is given as indicated for trunk, shoulders, shoulder girdle and head. The use of the head and shoulder girdle in flexion and rotation is essential in many functional activities, especially for patients with cervical or high thoracic lesions.

Caution As the fracture is recently healed, trunk mobilisation must be undertaken very gradually and with extreme care. Forced movements, particularly forced flexion, must be completely avoided. Initially only free active flexion is given.

PRELIMINARY TRAINING FOR FUNCTIONAL ACTIVITIES

Lifting the buttocks effectively by pushing on the arms is the basis of most of the activities of daily living. An effective lift depends upon balance and strength and upon knowing exactly where to place the hands and how to hold the head, shoulders and trunk. The following comments apply primarily to cervical and high thoracic lesions.

Where the abdominal muscles are innervated, trunk control will be adequate and all lifts will be relatively easy.

Basic principles

In order to maintain balance whilst moving, the first principle of body mechanics must be observed, that is, the line of gravity must remain inside the base of support. To achieve this in the sitting position with no muscle power around the hips, the head and shoulders must be kept forwards of the hip joints. When lifting the trunk with the hands just in front of the hip joints the head, trunk and hips *must be flexed as much as possible*. This position gives a mechanical advantage so that the same strength achieves a higher lift. An optimum degree of flexion will be reached beyond which the lift becomes impractical for those without triceps because the elbows will be flexed.

All patients start lifting themselves with extended elbows. Many patients *with* triceps later progress to lifting with the elbows flexed, when the mechanical advantage increases as the degree of hip flexion increases.

In all movements the head acts as a weight to assist or resist any movement. When the arms are short or when there is extra weight around the hips, lifting is more difficult (see Ch. 4).

The following manoeuvres provide the basis of functional activities such as dressing, turning in bed and transfers:

Lifting on the mat
Moving on the mat
Moving the paralysed limbs
Sitting up and lying down
Rolling prone and turning on to the side.

The therapist is behind, at the side or in front of the patient as required to assist or resist each component of the movements involved. Clear instructions should be given at every step. Initially assistance will be necessary to maintain sufficient flexion of the head and trunk as patients generally feel that they need to extend the trunk in order to lift. The therapist should never try to assist the patient in functional activities by lifting under the axillae. This action entirely negates any effort by the patient to lift by depressing the shoulders.

LIFTING ON THE MAT

The therapist

The therapist is behind the patient and, as well as maintaining the necessary flexion, may need to aid the lift with her hands under the buttocks. Later, where possible, stabilisations are given in the lifted position.

Action of the patient

1. To balance in long sitting, flex the head, shoulders and trunk so that the line of gravity is kept in front of the hip joints. With the arms close to the sides, place the hands on the mat slightly forward of the hips and preferably with the palms flat and fingers extended. Where triceps is paralysed lateral rotation of the arms assists stability at the elbows.

2. Lean forwards with the head and shoulders bent over the knees. A greater degree of flexion is needed by tetraplegic patients. When innervated the abdominal muscles will flex the trunk and the movement of the head and shoulders becomes less important.

3. With the elbows extended, push down on the hands.

4. *Depress the shoulders* and lift the buttocks off the mat. At the moment of lift raise the head. This will prevent the trunk collapsing forwards.

MOVING ON THE MAT

To lift sideways

The therapist

In addition to the factors already mentioned the therapist may need to encourage rotation.

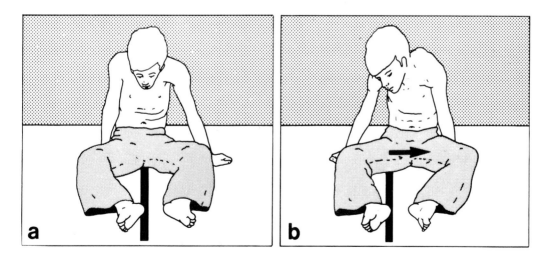

Fig. 9.1 Lifting sideways. Patient with a complete lesion below C_6 without triceps and with the clavicular portion of pectoralis major only.

Action of the patient

1. Place the right hand on the mat close to and slightly in front of the hip.

2. Place the left hand at the same level but approximately a foot away from the body. This distance will depend on the length of the arm in relation to that of the trunk. The elbows are extended and the forearms supinated, or in mid-position (Fig. 9.1a).

3. Flex further forwards over the knees and lift the buttocks. At the same time twist the head and shoulders to the right, bringing the left shoulder forwards and the right one back (Fig. 9.1b). Where latissimus dorsi is innervated it will pull the pelvis forwards towards the arm which is away from the side.

To lift forwards

The legs need to be in lateral rotation and free to flex at the knee.

1. Lean well forwards, with the head over the knees (Fig. 9.2).

2. Place the hands on the mat a little in front of the hip joints and close in to the sides. The elbows are extended and forearms supinated.

3. Lift the buttocks (Fig. 9.2b).

4. Keep the head flexed and the buttocks will move forwards. Once beyond the point of balance the patient will collapse forwards (Fig. 9.2).

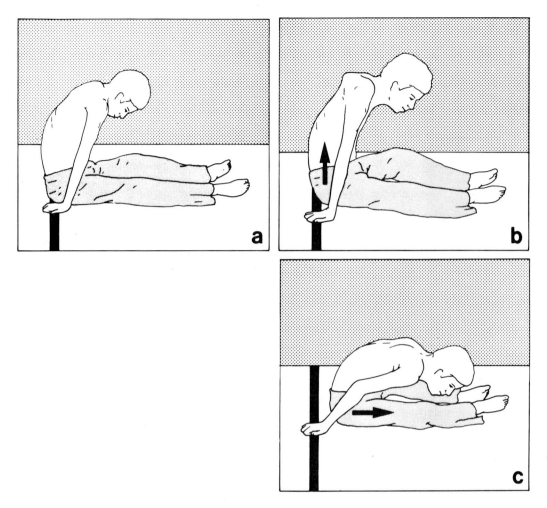

Fig. 9.2 Lifting forwards. Patient with a complete lesion below C$_6$ without triceps and with the clavicular portion of pectoralis major only.

MOVING THE PARALYSED LIMBS

In order to perform the activities of daily living the patient will need to lift and move his paralysed limbs.

The paraplegic patient will accomplish this quickly and easily, almost automatically. The tetraplegic patient will need intensive training and practice and must not be disheartened if success is delayed.

It is necessary to be able to:

1. Move the legs along the mat.
2. Cross one ankle over the other.
3. Cross one ankle over the opposite knee.
4. Flex the leg in sitting and side lying.

A method for tetraplegic patients to flex and lift the leg is described in the section 'To turn in bed' (p. 96).

Balance can be maintained whilst moving the legs by leaning forwards on one or both elbows. This position leaves the hands free to lift, push or pull the leg. The pelvis must be straight and the patient leans a little to one side, as well as forwards, to keep the body weight over the static leg.

SITTING AND LYING

To sit from the supine position without using a monkey pole

Action of the patient

Method 1

1. In one brisk movement throw the right arm over to the left, flex the head and shoulders and twist them to the left. This will rotate the upper part of the trunk (Fig. 9.3a and b).
2. Balance on both elbows (Fig. 9.3c).
3. Take the weight on the right elbow and bring the left elbow closer to the trunk.
4. Balance on the left elbow and, holding the head forwards and protracting the shoulders, transfer the right arm to the right side of the body and balance on both elbows (Fig. 9.3d).
5. Lean over on the left elbow, outwardly rotate the right arm and extend it behind the body (Fig. 9.3e). (Where possible step 4 can be omitted.)
6. Adjust the position until the weight can be taken on the right arm and extend the left arm in a similar manner (Fig. 9.3f).
7. Slowly bring the hands forwards alternately, a few inches at a time, until the weight is over the legs (Fig. 9.3g).

Method 2

1. With the arms in pronation by the sides put the wrists under the buttocks.
2. With the elbows on the mat strongly extend the wrists.
3. Flex the head, protract the shoulders, and with the elbows as the pivot-point pull the weight of the head and upper trunk onto the elbows.
4. Move each elbow backwards a few inches at a time.

Continue as in Method 1 steps 5, 6, and 7. If the patient finds difficulty with the hands under the hips, the thumbs can be hooked in the trouser pockets initially to enable the patient to get the feel of the movement.

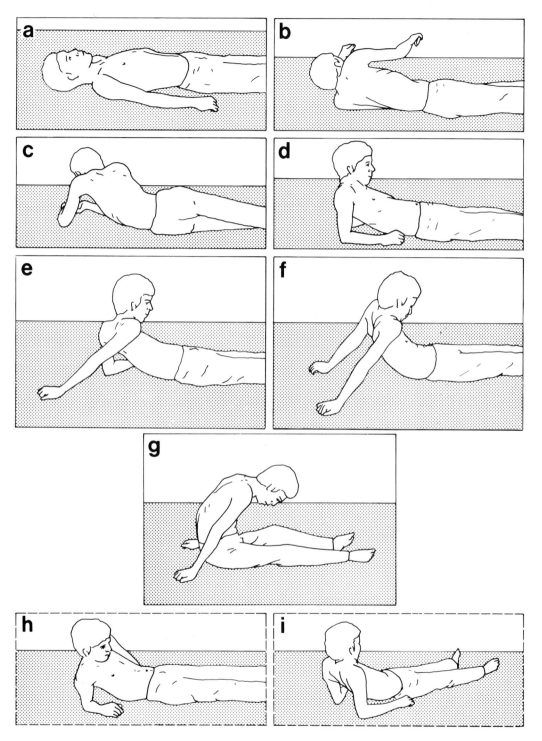

Fig. 9.3 (a–g) Sitting up. (h & i) Lying down. Patient with a complete lesion below C_6 without triceps and with the clavicular portion of pectoralis major only.

Method 3

From the position where the weight is on both elbows (Fig. 9.3c), the patient can 'walk' on his forearms along the mat to achieve the sitting position. Diagrams are given in Chapter 15.

To lie down from the sitting position

1. Keeping the head flexed and shoulders protracted, lean over to the right and drop the weight on to the right elbow (Fig. 9.3h).
2. Balance on the right elbow.
3. Flex the left arm and transfer half the weight on to the left elbow.
4. Still keeping the head and shoulders forwards (Fig. 9.3i), straighten one arm at a time until lying flat.

To sit from the supine position using a monkey pole

Position of the monkey pole

The point of suspension for the monkey pole is over the midline of the body, or slightly beyond midline towards the side of the supporting arm and approximately level with the xiphisternum. The handle should be just within the reach of the patient's extended wrist.

Action of the patient

To lift on to one elbow:

1. Extend the right arm and hook the extended wrist over the monkey pole (Fig. 9.4a).
2. Pull the body towards the monkey pole and lean on the left elbow (Fig. 9.4b).
3. Flex the right elbow over the monkey pole and hold the body weight, whilst bringing the left elbow closer to the trunk.
4. Support the body weight on the left elbow (Fig. 9.4c).

To get up on two extended arms, proceed with either of the following methods.

Method 1

5. Lean on the left elbow.
6. With the elbow flexed flick the right arm into lateral rotation and hold the wrist against the monkey pole chain (Fig. 9.4d).
7. Hold the body weight with the right arm, outwardly rotate the left shoulder and extend the arm behind the body (Fig. 9.4e).

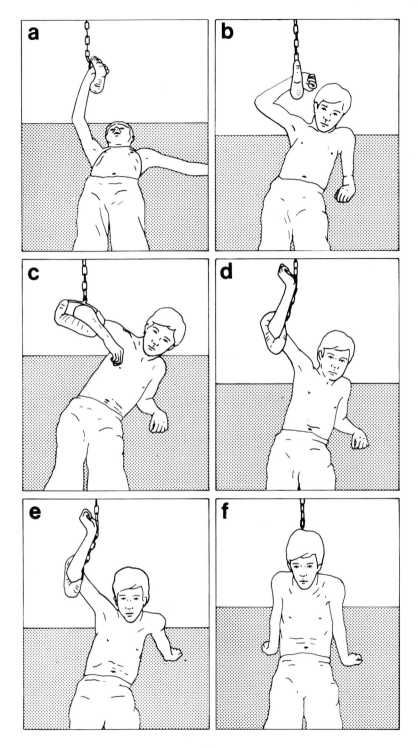

Fig. 9.4 Sitting up using a monkey pole. Patient with a complete lesion below C$_6$ without triceps and with the clavicular portion of pectoralis major only.

8. Lean well over the left arm, release the monkey pole and extend the right arm behind the body.

9. Move the hands forwards alternately, a few inches at a time, until the weight is over the legs (Fig. 9.4f).

Method 2

5. Lean well over to the left and balance on left elbow.

6. Take the right arm out of the monkey pole, outwardly rotate the shoulder, and extend the arm behind the body.

7. Transfer most of the weight on to the right arm and push the left arm straight.

8. Move the hands forwards alternately, a few inches at a time until the weight is over the legs.

Patients without pectoral muscles or with the clavicular head of pectoralis major only, may find Method 1 the easier. Patients with good hand function grasp the monkey pole with one hand and lift on to the opposite elbow. From there the procedure is the same as Method 2.

Occasionally a paraplegic patient may need to use a monkey pole for one of the following reasons: age, overweight, ossification around the hip joints or a previous medical history of heart or lung disease.

To roll prone from the supine position

Action of the patient

To roll to the right:

1. Flex the head and shoulders and fling the arms over to the left, so that the necessary momentum can be gained in stage 2 (Fig. 9.5a).

2. In one brisk movement flex the head and shoulders and fling the arms from left to right. As this movement is completed the right shoulder is pulled back as far as possible (Fig. 9.5b).

3. The momentum of the arms is transferred to the trunk and legs and the lower half of the body will roll prone (Fig. 9.5c).

4. Place the left forearm on the mat and take the weight on it.

5. Pull the right shoulder back and take the weight on both forearms (Fig. 9.5d).

6. Lie flat and put the arms by the sides.

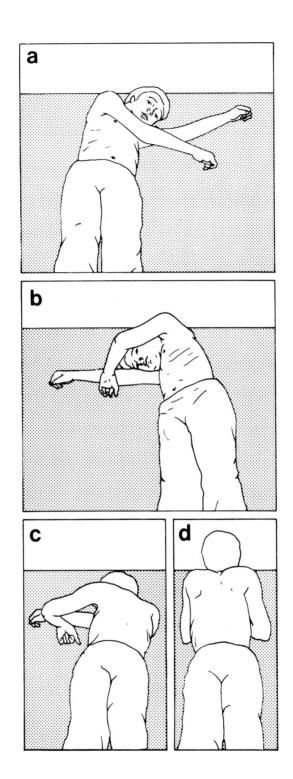

Fig. 9.5 Rolling. Patient with a complete lesion below C_6 without triceps and with the clavicular portion of pectoralis major only.

To turn on to the side

Action of the patient

1. Sit up with or without the monkey pole as described.
2. Lean on the left extended arm.
3. Hook the extended right wrist under the right knee and flex the leg.
4. Facing the left, lean down on the left elbow and at the same time pull the right leg into further flexion and cross the right knee over the left leg.
5. Place the right forearm on the mat and take the weight on it.
6. Lower the trunk into side lying.

To turn in bed

When the patient is able to turn on the mat and to move and position his legs, progression is made to turning in bed.

Action of the patient

The patient turns from supine to right side lying and must position the leg pillow.

To sit up, either of the two ways already described can be used, or the patient can sit up using a bed loop. The loop is attached to the end of the bed and is just long enough to hook on the forearm.

1. Put the left forearm through the loop and flex the right elbow extending the wrist to 'grip' the edge of the mattress (Fig. 9.6a).
2. Pull on the loop with the left arm; and transfer the weight onto the right elbow (Fig. 9.6b).
3. Release the strap (Fig. 9.6c).
4. Extend the left arm behind the body and take the weight on it (Fig. 9.6d).
5. Extending the right arm, take the weight on both arms. Move the hands forwards until the weight is over the legs (Fig. 9.6e).

To position the pillow:

6. Flex the left knee with the extended left wrist and push the pillow under the knee (Fig. 9.6f).

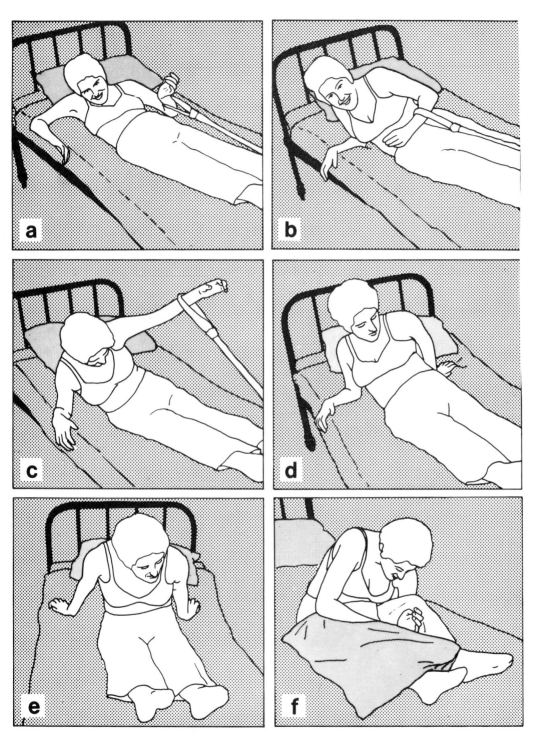

Fig. 9.6 Turning in bed. Patient with a complete lesion below C_7 with wrist control only.

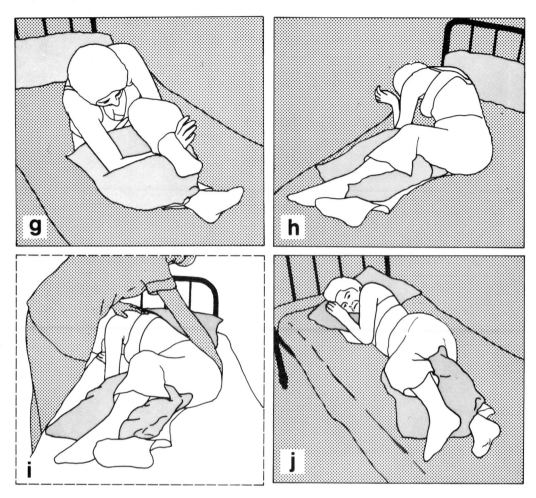

Fig. 9.6 (contd)

7. Keeping the weight well over the right hip, lift the lower leg on to the pillow with the right arm (Fig. 9.6g).
Adjust the position of the pillow and legs.

8. Turn the upper trunk to the right and take the weight firstly on the right and then on both elbows.

9. Lean forwards and take the maximum weight on the left elbow and forearm. Rock onto the left elbow and pivot the buttocks backwards across the bed (Fig. 9.6h).

10. When adequate movement backwards has been achieved, adjust the head pillow for individual comfort.

11. Take the weight onto the left elbow and lower the weight onto the right shoulder lying down on the side (Fig. 9.6j).

Initially the therapist may need to assist the patient to achieve the rocking movement by pressing down over the patient's left shoulder girdle with one hand and lifting under the right buttock with the other (Fig. 9.6i).

Group mat activities

Group activity is very useful, even though some patients may need individual assistance. Patients can watch and copy others with similar lesions accomplishing the various manoeuvres.

Competitive exercises using balls, bean bags, or balloons improve sitting balance and co-ordination.

Paraplegic patients can enjoy weight training in a group, and competitive exercise with heavier equipment can also be useful.

10

Wheelchairs and wheelchair management

TYPES OF WHEELCHAIR

Hand-propelled folding transit chair: standard and junior models

Most firms make the two main sizes of wheelchairs: standard (or adult) and junior. The difference between these is usually 2 inches in seat width and 2 inches in overall height. There is very little difference in weight. In general there are also two sizes for children. It is often possible to put a larger seat and backrest on to the largest of the children's chairs to adapt for the growing child. On all chairs the foot rests need to be swinging and detachable to allow easy access for transfers. For the same reason the armrests need to be detachable.

The angle of incline of the backrest should not be more than 5°. The diameter of the wheels varies from 18–24 inches. The larger the wheels the less effort involved in pushing the chair. The 8-inch casters are preferred to the 5-inch, as they are easier to push over carpets, kerbs and other small obstacles.

Wheels

Large wheels at the back and small ones at the front allow the patient to remain supported by the backrest whilst pushing the chair.

Pneumatic rear and solid front tyres give the best combination for function and comfort.

Pneumatic front tyres are used when the patient's predominant need is to push over rough ground. They give less vibration but are harder to push.

Footplates

The footplates need either heel loops or a calf strap to prevent the feet slipping backwards off the footplates and becoming entangled with the front wheels. Heel loops are easier if the footplates are constantly being removed for transfers, etc. If the patient is excessively spastic in the lower limbs both may be necessary.

The approximate weight of the standard chair is 54 lb (25 kg).

The lightweight chair

A lightweight chair is made by most firms in the standard models. It is approximately two-thirds of the weight of the standard model. Some patients who are constantly putting the chair into a car prefer this type.

Exceptionally lightweight chairs are available with a forward folding mechanism, multi-variant frame and wheels which can be detached for easy transport.

A semi-reclining back chair

A wheelchair in which the backrest can be angled to 30° from the vertical is made by several firms. This chair allows patients with high cervical lesions to balance and breathe more easily. It is obviously heavier than the standard model and the overall length is greater, making it more difficult to manoeuvre in a small area. This chair is commonly used for the ultra-high lesion.

The transit chair

This chair is attendant-propelled, having small wheels at the front and rear. It is approximately the weight of the lightweight chair. It is a necessity for the patient using a power-drive chair and useful for the patient with a semi-reclining chair. The various components of the power-drive chair are heavy, and it is time-consuming to dismantle it for transport.

The power-drive chair

The power-drive chair is manufactured in both standard and junior sizes. There are three means of control:

1. arm or hand control
2. breath control
3. chin control.

The weight of the chair with the batteries is approximately double the weight of the standard chair. It is used by patients who are unable to push a wheelchair.

The stand-up chair

This chair enables the patient to raise himself to the standing position to perform an activity and to sit down again independently. The seat of the chair is raised slowly to the required height by pressing a simple switch. The movement can be interrupted or reversed at will.

The chair with variable seat height

Some firms manufacture a chair in which the seat, with backrest, footrests, and armrests, can be raised 10 inches.

Wheelchair accessories

There are various accessories which can be obtained with most models when necessary.

Armrests

There are three models; all detachable:

1. standard
2. desk arms — the front upper quarter is cut away to allow the chair to be wheeled closer to a desk or table
3. adjustable.

Most detachable armrests have automatic locking devices.

Brake extensions

These are sometimes necessary to enable patients with cervical lesions to reach the brakes without falling forwards.

Capstans

Capstans are rubber capped projections spaced at regular intervals around the rim of the wheel. These help some patients with high cervical lesions to get a purchase on the wheels when pushing the chair.

Crutch or walking stick holder

This consists of a small platform attached to the tipping lever and a strap on the upper part of the backrest to carry the crutches.

Elevating leg rests

These increase the overall length of the chair by 4–5 inches and its weight by approximately 2 pounds. They are useful for:

1. patients with high lesions with vasomotor problems
2. any patient with a leg injury
3. a tall patient with long legs where elevation allows floor clearance, especially over rough ground.

Easy transfer wheelchair attachment

This device consists of two parts, either or both of which can be fitted to most chairs with removable armrests. The major part enables the rear wheel on one side to be moved backwards to facilitate transfers. The second part is an armrest which converts to a sliding board with backrest.

Footplate angle adjustments

These permit the selection of the most comfortable angle of the footplate for the user.

Head extension

This can be attached to the backrest to increase its height and give added support when necessary.

Kerb climber

This device enables kerbs of up to 5 inches to be mounted in a power-drive chair.

Mobile arm support

A splint supports the weight of the arm and pivots allow maximum performance from minimum motor power.

No-mor flats

The inner tube of a standard tyre is replaced by one made of a rubber compound with a hollow core. This is puncture proof and does not need to be inflated. It provides a comfortable ride, and is useful if propelling over rough ground, but it increases the weight of the chair and should not be fitted if a lightweight chair is essential.

Restraining or safety strap

This is attached to the supports for the backrest on each side and fastens with velcro across the abdomen. All patients with cervical lesions use them when first mobile, and those with lesions at C_{4-5} and above continue to use them.

Tray

The tray clips on to the armrests and provides a useful surface for many activities. It is also useful, when well padded, as a support for the arms for patients with high cervical lesions.

Wheelchair narrower

This can be fixed to the frame of the wheelchair. It will reduce the width of the chair by about 4 inches and permit the chair to pass through narrow doorways.

Zipper backrest

This can be fitted to standard and junior chairs and permits entry and exit from the rear of the chair.

THE POSITION OF THE PATIENT IN THE WHEELCHAIR

The majority of patients are apprehensive and unstable when first sitting up in a wheelchair. They are unwilling to release their grasp on the armrests and sit afraid to move. Gradually the patient becomes adjusted and learns to relax in the chair. This can only occur if:

    a. the chair is a suitable type for the patient, and
    b. if it is adjusted to support him correctly.

The following questions itemise the points the therapist should look for to ensure adequate support and safety. The questions are applicable to most transit chairs in current use. (Fig. 10.1)

Seat

1. Is the patient sitting on a suitable (e.g. 4 inch Dunlopillo) cushion to avoid excessive pressure?

2. *Width.* To avoid pressure on the hips is there the space of two fingers' breadth each side between the patient and the armrest? Alternatively is the seat so wide that the patient finds difficulty in reaching the wheels comfortably?

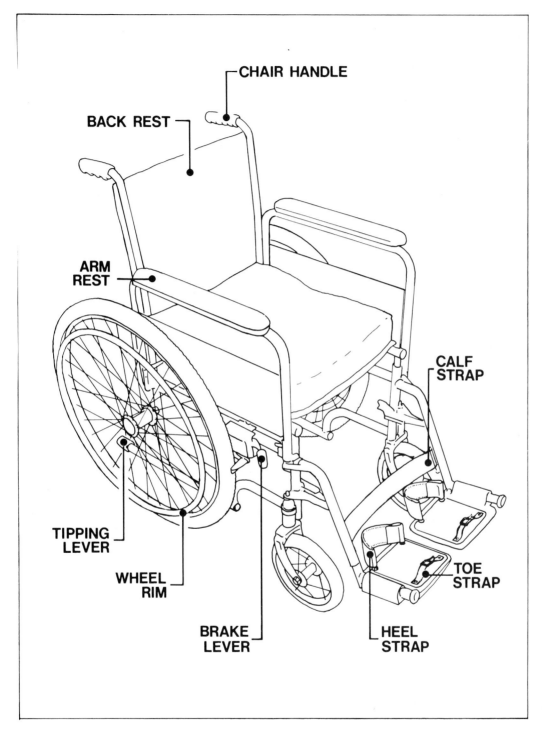

Fig. 10.1 Various wheelchair components and accessories.

3. *Depth.* Is the patient sitting *upright* in the chair with his weight on the ischii and well supported by the back rest at an angle of 90°? Or is the seat too deep and the weight consequently on the sacrum? This can be the case for children, and for adults with short legs. If a less deep seat is not available a small upright cushion can be placed behind the patient.

Footplates

1. Are the footplates the correct height so that the thighs are completely supported?

If the knees are higher than the hips, excessive pressure is thrown on to the ischii and if the patient wears a urinal the urine will not drain adequately. If the knees are lower than the hips, the patient may slip forwards out of the chair. This particularly applies to those with severe spasticity in the hip extensor muscles. As the weight will be on the toes the spasticity will be increased.

2. Are toe straps needed to hold the feet down against dorsiflexor or extensor spasticity?

Toe straps can be potentially dangerous for some active, young patients with extreme spasticity in the hip extensors. With the feet held down, a spasm may throw the patient out of the chair. A padded strap in front of the knees may be useful to hold such a patient back in the chair.

Backrest

1. Is the backrest too high so that it prevents the patient flexing his elbow round the chair handle for support?

2. Is it too low so that the patient leans back over it? If it is too low will it be satisfactory once the patient has learnt to balance and flex his spine? In this case a temporary extension may be all that is necessary for a week or two.

3. Does the patient need a small cushion in the lumbar region to extend the lumbar spine when sitting? This is often necessary for children and patients with lesions above T_5 where a long 'C' curve often develops.

4. Is there any area on the patient's back which might take too large a share of pressure and become a sore, i.e., prominent spines, a dubus, scoliosis, old scar? Padding of foam rubber or orthopaedic felt can be attached to the chair on either side of the potentially dangerous area to relieve it of any pressure.

Armrests

1. With the shoulders relaxed do the forearms rest comfortably on

the standard armrests? If the patient is short or exceptionally tall are adjustable armrests required? Has the patient a high, unequal lesion, e.g. C_{4-5}, and needs armrests of different height on each side so that the weaker side has adequate support?

2. Does the patient need desk arms as well as or instead of, full armrests to use at desk and tables? Will desk arms give sufficient support if the patient needs to lean on his forearms to balance? All but very low lesions need full armrests initially.

3. If there is a lever for locking the armrests into position, can the patient manage to manipulate it? If not, will he do so in time, with further practise?

Brakes

1. Can the patient reach the brakes? If the patient has a cervical lesion are brake extensions necessary?

Waist strap

1. Does the patient need a restraining strap round the waist?

All tetraplegic patients should use one until balance in sitting is achieved. Patients with lesions C_{3-4} and C_{4-5} should always wear one for safety.

Wedge between knees

1. Does the patient have adductor spasticity and need a wedge between the knees to prevent the development of pressure sores?

The wedge, or 'dolly', should be made large enough to keep the thighs abducted and so weaken the adductor stretch reflex.

The core of the wedge can be made of old blanket or other firm material, but this should be covered overall with thick foam rubber and encased in stockinette.

COUGHING IN A WHEELCHAIR

Unassisted coughing

To cough unaided the patient must himself produce the pressure usually given by the abdominal muscles.
This can be done in the following ways:

1. Hold one armrest, press the other arm against the abdomen and lean well over it.

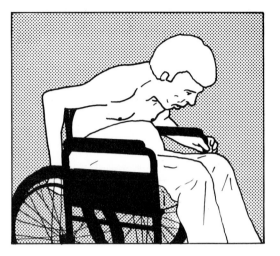

Fig. 10.2 Independent coughing in patient with a complete lesion below C_6.

2. Flex one elbow behind the chairback or chair handle, press the other arm against the abdomen and lean over it.

3. Hold both armrests or flex the elbows behind the chair handles and lean well over until the chest is pressing against the thighs (or abdomen if large) (Fig. 10.2).

To assist a patient to cough in a wheelchair

The methods on page 40 can be used.

For the ultra-high lesion, e.g. the patient with a lesion at C_4 with a partially paralysed diaphragm, the following method is useful.

The *first therapist* stands behind the chair and, linking her hands in front of the patient, pulls back against the upper abdominal wall and lower ribs.

The *second therapist* stands in front of the patient and pushes on the upper thorax.

WHEELCHAIR MANOEUVRES

The basic movements within the wheelchair and the initial wheelchair manoeuvres are written for *tetraplegic patients without a grip*. The basic safety measures, such as holding on with one elbow or wrist, become progressively unnecessary as the level of the lesion descends. The advanced wheelchair manoeuvres are divided into sections, since some activities are unsuitable for patients with cervical lesions. Adaptions in technique may have to be made for chairs with minor differences in construction, for example, in the type of brake lever.

Basic movements within the wheelchair

1. To manipulate the brakes.
2. To remove the armrest.
3. To pick up objects from the floor.
4. To reach down to the footplates.
5. To lift the buttocks forwards in the chair.

Whenever the patient prepares to move within the wheelchair or to move into or out of it, he must first give attention to the position of the wheelchair itself.

To give maximum stability, the small front wheels must point forwards, as this prevents the chair tipping on to the footplates, and the brakes must be on. If the patient is going to lean out of the chair in any direction the buttocks must be well back in the seat.

1. To manipulate the brakes

To reach the right brake:

1. Hook the left elbow behind the left chair handle.
2. Lean forwards and to the right allowing the left biceps to lengthen as the trunk movement occurs.

To release the brake use flexion of the elbow and shoulder to push the lever forwards with the palm of the hand or the lower part of the supinated forearm (Fig. 10.3a). To apply the brake, pull the lever back using the right biceps and either the extended wrist (lesion at C_6) (Fig. 10.3b), or the supinated forearm (lesion at C_5).

2. To remove the right armrest

1. To release the catch push down with the base of the thumb over the catch (Fig. 10.3c).
2. Hook the right elbow behind the right chair handle.
3. Place the left hand at the front and the right hand at the back of the right armrest. Using the wrist extension grip lift the armrest out of its sockets with both hands (Fig. 10.3d).
4. Hold the armrest with the left hand and balance it on the supinated forearm (Fig. 10.3e).
5. Place the armrest on the floor beside the rear wheel, or hook it over the left chair handle.

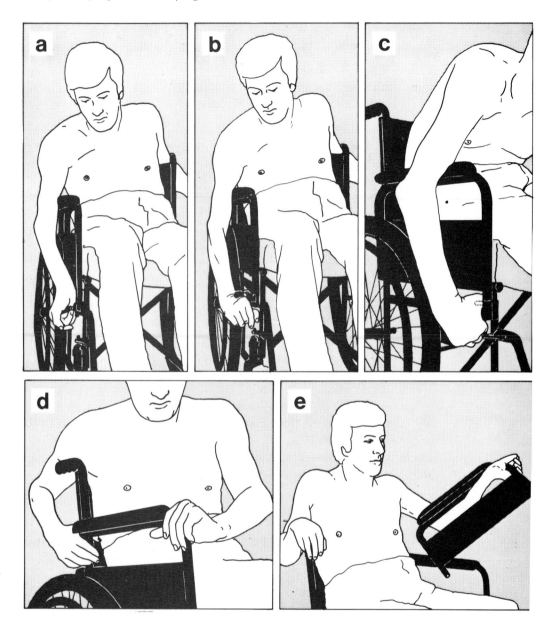

Fig. 10.3 (a & b) Manipulating the brakes. (c, d & e) Removing the armrest. Patient with a complete lesion below C_6 without triceps.

3. To pick up objects from the floor

Objects are picked up by leaning sideways out of the chair and not by leaning forwards over the footplates; the forwards position is unstable and therefore dangerous.

To lean to the left

Position the chair sideways on to the object. Hook the right elbow behind the right chair handle and lean over the left armrest. To avoid excessive pressure on the rib cage, maintain this position for only a few seconds at a time. The armrest can be removed to allow shorter patients the necessary reach.

To regain the upright position pull up with the right elbow. When triceps is innervated the extended wrist can be used under the outer rim of the armrest to maintain balance and regain the upright position.

4. To reach down to the footplates

This position will be necessary to fasten the toe straps, adjust the footplates, empty the urinal or for adjustments when dressing.

1. Lean forwards on the elbows on the armrests.
2. Change the position of the arms one by one and lean on the forearms on the thighs.
3. Put one hand at a time down to the feet leaning the chest on the thighs.

To regain the upright position

Patients without triceps must (a) throw the stronger arm back over the backrest and hook the extended wrist behind the chair handle, and (b) pull the trunk upright by strongly extending the wrist and flexing the elbow.

Patients with good functioning triceps pull the trunk upright by hooking one or both extended wrist(s) underneath the upper, outer edge of the armrest(s).

5. To lift the buttocks forward in the chair

Patients with cervical lesions without triceps

This manoeuvre is described in detail in Chapter 10, page 126.

Patients with cervical lesions with triceps

To lift the right buttock forwards:

　1. Lean over the left forearm, which is placed well forwards on the armrest.
　2. Lift on the right hand on the armrest.
　3. At the same time throw the head back and wriggle the right buttock forward (Fig. 10.4).

Repeat to lift the left buttock forward.

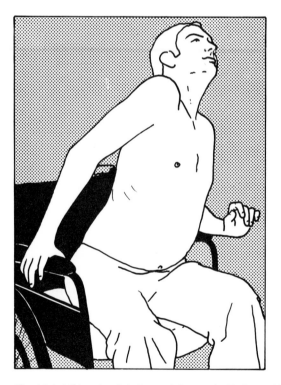

Fig. 10.4 Lifting the right buttock forwards. Patient with a complete lesion below C_7 with wrist control only.

Patients with Paraplegia

1. Lift on both armrests.
2. Extend the head and shoulders and 'throw' the buttocks forward.

Initial and advanced wheelchair manoeuvres

When putting the wheelchair in motion in any direction the position of the head and shoulders is important. They are used to reinforce the action of the arms, whether to gain greater momentum or to act as a brake.

Many patients start moving the chair by pushing on the tyres. Paraplegic patients usually progress to using the wheel rims, but many patients with tetraplegia continue to use the tyres because they find the purchase easier and the push more effective. Pushing gloves are used by tetraplegic patients to protect the skin from callous formation and abrasions due to friction or injury (Fig. 8.1d).

Patients with lesions at C_{4-5} try to push the wheelchair using temporary capstans on the wheels. Although most patients at this level will need a power-drive chair for permanent use at home, excellent exercise is provided by attempting to push on the uncarpeted floors of the hospital. Small pieces of adhesive felt can be bound onto the rim at suitable intervals with adhesive tape. Temporary capstans may help older patients with lesions at C_5 to learn to push the chair.

Initial wheelchair manoeuvres

1. To push on the flat.
2. To use the chair on sloping ground.
3. To turn the chair.

1. To push on the flat

When wheeling on the flat the push forwards with the arms is reinforced if accompanied by strong flexion of the head and shoulder girdle. Momentum is gained because there is a general thrust forward with the upper part of the body.

To reverse on the flat

1. Put both arms over the backrest between the chair handles.
2. Place the hands on the wheels with the elbows extended and shoulders elevated.
3. Leaning backwards, depress the shoulders and thrust downwards, with as much weight as possible over the arms. Slopes can be ascended in reverse in this way if the patient is unable to push up forwards.

2. To use the chair on sloping ground

To push up a slope:
1. Leaning forward, place the hands towards the back of the top of the tyre (Fig. 10.5a).
2. Push forwards using flexion of the elbows and flexion and adduction of the shoulders (Fig. 10.5b). The chair can be held on a slope by turning the wheels across the incline.
To slow down when going down a slope:
Extend the head and shoulders and brake either with both hands towards the front of the tyres or with the first metacarpals under the wheel rims and the wrists extended (Fig. 10.5c).

3. To turn the wheelchair to right

1. Place the right hand towards the back of the tyre with the arm over the back rest, behind the chair handle.
2. Laterally rotate the right arm and with the body weight over the hand push backwards on the inner side of the wheel (Fig. 10.5d).
3. Push forwards with the left hand.

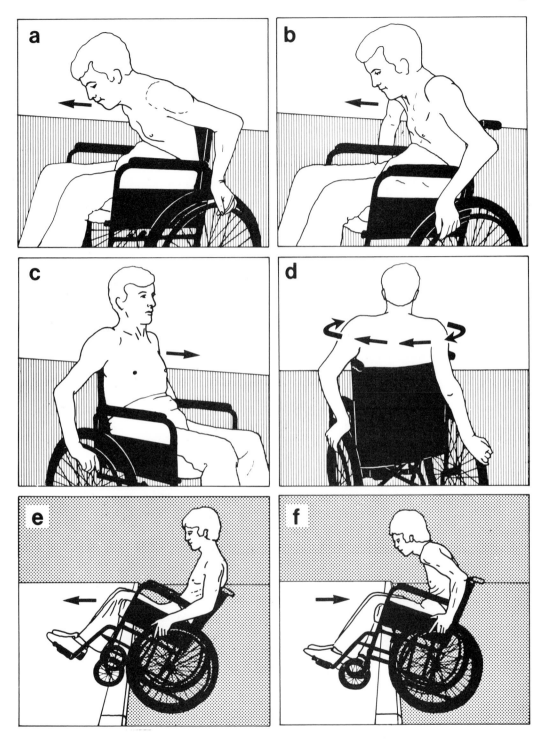

Fig. 10.5 (a & b) Pushing up a slope. (c) Pushing down a slope. (d) Turning.
(e) Pushing up a kerb. (f) Descending a kerb. (a–d) Patient with a complete lesion
below C_6 without triceps. (e & f) Patient with a complete lesion below T_8.

Advanced wheelchair manoeuvres: Tetraplegic patients

1. To push the chair over a 2-inch step

This manoeuvre can be accomplished by patients with lesions at C_6 without triceps and may be necessary to get over a draft excluder or similar obstacle.

1. Place the palms on top and to the outer side of the tyre with the fingers down over the rim and the thumb between the rim and the tyre.
2. Push the chair backwards, then
3. Push briskly forwards leaning the body weight forward at the same time.

Advanced wheelchair manoeuvres: Paraplegic patients

1. To mount and descend a kerb.
2. To balance on the rear wheels.
3. To 'jump' the chair sideways.
4. To transfer a wheelchair into a car.

1. To mount and descend a kerb

This activity can be accomplished by patients with a normal grip, that is, those with lesions at T_1 and below.

To push up a kerb

1. Tilt the chair onto the rear wheels.
2. Push forwards until the front wheels hang over the kerb (Fig. 10.5e) and lower them gently.
3. Leaning forward, push forwards forcefully to bring the rear wheels on to the pavement.

If the patient is unable to tilt the chair onto the rear wheels, he should 'flick' the front wheels high enough to mount the kerb. The flick up is achieved in the same way as the tilt but requires less strength and balance. Patients with lesions at C_{7-8} with good hand function may mount kerbs in this way.

To descend a kerb

With the back to the kerb, lean well forward and push slowly backwards until the rear and then the front wheels roll down the kerb (Fig. 10.5f).

2. Rear wheel balance

Balance and movement on the rear wheels is useful to facilitate independent travel over rough ground, for example over grass, sand or shale, and also in negotiating kerbs or a step.

This technique is safe only for patients with a good grip, that is, for patients with lesions at T_1 and below.

There are three manoeuvres involved:

1. To tilt the chair onto the rear wheels.
2. To balance the chair on the rear wheels.
3. To move and turn the chair on the rear wheels.

The therapist

The therapist always stands behind the patient in step standing with the thigh of the forward leg ready to support the chair if control is lost. She holds the chair handles loosely (Fig. 10.6d).

Assistance is given to tilt the chair by pressing down on the chair handles, and to find the balance point by giving pressure in each direction as necessary.

The therapist's hands must be very sensitive to the movement of the chair, correcting it only when the patient is out of control. She must allow enough scope for the patient to be really aware of each movement that occurs, so that the patient can become familiar with the 'feel' of the chair in the balance position.

Caution *The therapist's hands must remain on the chair handles until the patient has complete control, as it is all too easy for the patient to overbalance backwards and injure himself. Much practice will be needed. Not until the therapist is entirely satisfied that the patient is utterly competent should he be allowed to balance without her behind him as a safeguard.*

The action of the patient

To tilt the chair onto the rear wheels

1. Place the hands on the wheels approximately in the 10 o'clock position, holding the tyre and the rim.
2. Slightly extend the head and
3. Put pressure on the wheels as though moving backwards (Fig. 10.6a).
4. Push forwards quickly and forcefully, and the front wheels will lift off the floor (Fig. 10.6b).

The height of the lift depends upon the force of the push.

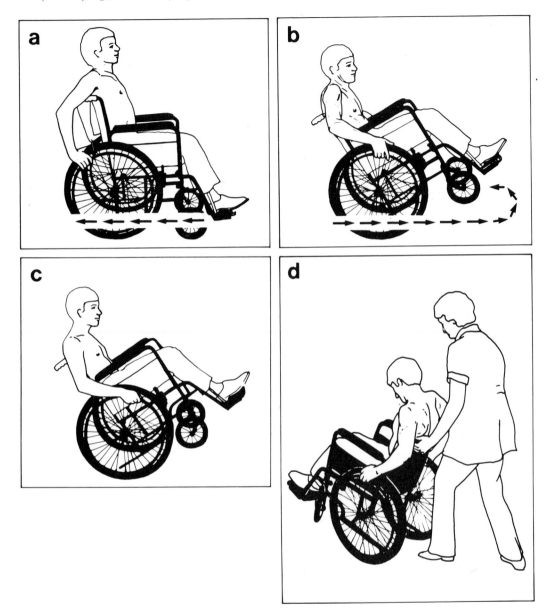

Fig. 10.6 Rear wheel balance.

To balance on the rear wheels

The balance point is much further back than most patients realise. It is found by playing the wheels forwards and backwards and using the head and shoulders as a counter-weight. When overbalancing forwards push the wheels forwards. When overbalancing backwards push the wheels backwards. Control is usually easier when holding the rims and not the wheels (Fig. 10.6c).

To move and turn on the rear wheels

Once balance is achieved it is not difficult to move on the rear wheels. The technique is the same as with the front wheels down.

3. To 'jump' the chair sideways

This manoeuvre can be useful when turning into a doorway from a narrow passage.

1. Apply the brakes.
2. Lean away from the back of the chair.
3. Grip the highest point of the wheel rims.
4. Lift the buttocks off the chair and
5. Quickly lift the wheels up and sideways before the buttocks descend again to the seat.

4. To transfer the wheelchair into a car

Patients can transfer the wheelchair into the car through the front passenger door. The chair is accommodated either in front of or behind the seat, which is adjusted accordingly.

Method 1

1. Transfer into the car through the passenger door.
2. Fold the wheelchair, leaving the brakes off.
3. Lift the front wheels of the chair into the car.
4. Transfer to the driver's seat.
5. Pull the chair into the car.

Method 2

Alternatively, after step 2 of method 1:

3. Transfer to the driver's seat.
4. Lean across the passenger seat and tip the chair onto its rear wheels.
5. Pull the chair, rear wheels first, into the car.

The efficiency of either method largely depends upon the physical proportions of the patient, and the best way should be found by trial and error. To get the chair out of the car the procedure is reversed. It is easier to push the chair out when the rear wheels are adjacent to the door, that is, using Method 1.

11

Transfers

For patients with spinal cord injury transfers fall broadly into three groups:

   1. Those in which the feet are lifted and the trunk moves horizontally, e.g. transfer to plinth or bed.

   2. Those in which the feet are at floor level and the trunk moves horizontally, e.g. transfer to toilet or easy chair.

   3. Those in which the feet remain on the floor and the trunk moves vertically, e.g. transfer to bath or floor.

The first group is the most stable. The second requires skilled balance. The third requires considerable strength.

These factors explain the division of the transfers into *initial* and *advanced* for both tetraplegic and paraplegic patients. All patients commence with the transfers in group 1. Tetraplegic patients *without triceps* progress only to the easiest of those in group 2. As can be seen in the following list, advanced transfers for the most active tetraplegic with triceps and wrist control only reach group 3 with the bath transfer, whereas advanced transfers for paraplegic patients are in group 3 exclusively:

For patients with tetraplegia

Initial transfers: Chair to plinth
                        Removal of footplates
Advanced transfers: Chair to bed
                        Chair to car
                        Chair to toilet
                        Chair to easy chair } for patients with triceps
                        Chair to bath

For patients with paraplegia

Initial transfers: Chair to plinth or bed, sideways and forwards

Chair to car
Chair to toilet, sideways and backwards
Chair to easy chair
Advanced transfers: Chair to bath
Chair to floor

TECHNIQUE

The techniques described are those most commonly used for the various transfers. Slight variations will occur depending upon the individual height, weight, agility, and age of the patient and the level of the lesion.

All transfers except for that from the chair to the floor are described for the tetraplegic patient. It is a simple matter to adapt the transfer for a patient with a lower lesion. The patient is always to *lift* and not drag his body and to avoid knocking his limbs on the furniture or his buttocks on the wheel.

Whilst transferring the buttocks, the head, shoulders and trunk must be flexed with the head well forwards over the knees. It is *essential* that the plinth be the same height as the wheelchair for transfer training, and, ideally, all surfaces should be the correct height. Tetraplegic patients will achieve a transfer only under these conditions, but after training, most paraplegic patients will transfer to any surface without difficulty.

The Chair

In all cases the chair must be in the position of maximum stability. It may slip daring the transfer if the tyres are worn or the floor slippery, or if the patient pushes horizontally instead of vertically.

The footplates are removed except for independent transfer to the plinth or bed. It is dangerous only to pull up the footplates without swinging them out, since they may catch on the malleolii, and cause bruising or damage to the skin.

TRANSFERS BY THE THERAPIST

1. The 'cervical lift' using two therapists

This lift is used to transfer a patient to and from the plinth, bed, floor or second chair.

Transfer from bed to chair

Position of the chair

The chair is angled at approximately 30° to the side of the bed.

Position of the patient

The patient is in long sitting with the head and trunk flexed and with the arms folded across the lower ribs.

Position of the therapists to transfer the patient to the left

Operator number 1 stands behind the patient with one leg each side of the right rear wheel. She holds the patient round the thorax grasping the folded arms (as described in Ch. 7). The therapist must grip the *lower* thorax with her forearms to prevent the upper spine from elongating as the patient is lifted.

Operator number 2 is in step standing facing the bed. She grasps the legs with one arm high up under the thighs and the other under the lower legs. The heavier the patient the higher up the legs the grasp needs to be (Fig. 11.1a).

On a prearranged signal both operators lift together, number 1 taking a step sideways and number 2 a step backwards. The patient must be lifted high enough to avoid knocking the buttocks against the rear wheel or the spine against the chair handle or backrest support (Fig. 11.1b).

2. The transfer through standing using one therapist

This method is used to transfer a tetraplegic patient who can give little or no assistance.

Position of the patient

1. Bring the buttocks forwards in the chair until the feet are on the floor.

2. Flex the trunk and hips until the patient can 'hold' onto the therapist's shoulder with his chin.

3. If biceps is innervated hold round the therapist's neck. If the arms are completely paralysed they hang in front of the knees.

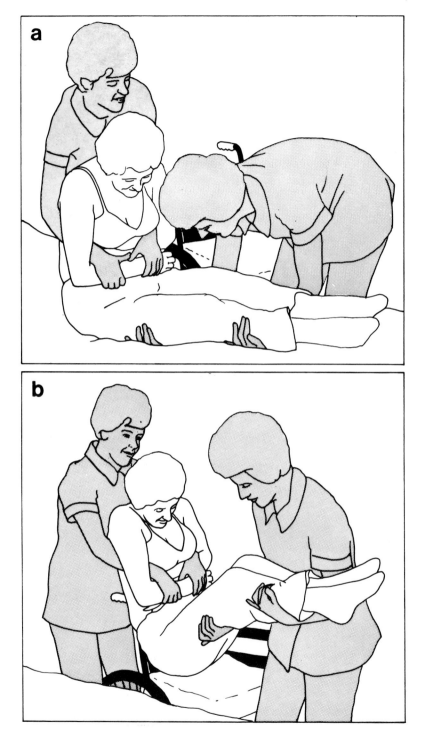

Fig. 11.1 Transferring a tetraplegic patient.

The therapist

1. Brace the feet and knees against the outside of the patient's feet and knees. Turn the feet in to 'hold' the patient's heels and maintain their position should a flexor spasm occur at the knees.
2. Flex the hips, keep the back straight and hold the patient under the buttocks. If the patient is overweight or is unable to grip with his chin, it may be necessary to grasp the trousers or trouser band. This should be avoided where possible, because the pull of the trousers may cause skin damage.
3. The head is turned either to one side or, when necessary, the chin grips the patient's shoulder (Fig. 11.2a).

To stand up

1. Lock the patient's feet and knees.
2. Keep the back straight.
3. Lean the body weight backwards to counterbalance the patient's weight, and at the same time,
4. Rock the patient against the knees and pull him into standing. Depending upon the relative sizes of the patient and the therapist a step back with one foot may be necessary to maintain balance. Control must be kept of the patient's legs.

To turn round

1. Extend the back and
2. Pivot the patient round to the therapist's left, with the weight of the patient taken through the therapist's trunk. (Fig. 11.2b).
(Notice the feet have knocked the right front wheel during the turn. Also the patient's left leg has spasmed into extension at the knee, but the therapist still has control of it.)

To sit down

1. Flex the hips and
2. Adjust the position of the hands. Either the left hand remains under the buttocks and the right hand slides up over the scapula, or both hands slide up the back to the scapula region to control the thorax.
3. At the same time, keeping control with the knees, allow the patient to flex at the hips and
4. Gently lower the buttocks to the seat (Fig. 11.2c).

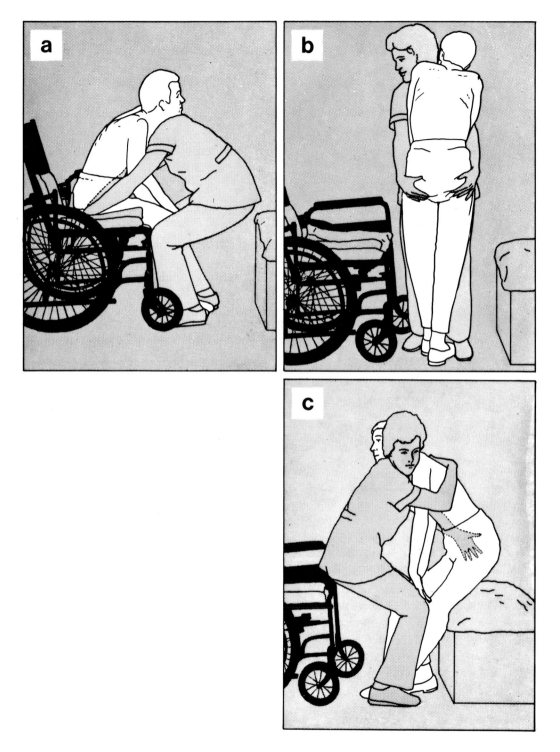

Fig. 11.2 Transfer through standing. Patient with a complete lesion below C₄.

INDEPENDENT TRANSFERS

To transfer to the plinth (moving to the right)

This transfer consists of three manoeuvres:

1. To bring the buttocks forwards in the chair.
2. To lift the legs onto the plinth.
3. To transfer the trunk.

Position of the chair

Line the chair up with the plinth at an approximate angle of 20°. With the buttocks forward in the chair, this small angle allows the transfer to occur in front of the rear wheel. A pillow is placed over the rear wheel to prevent injury should the buttocks knock against it during training.

The therapist

The therapist stands in front of the patient, ready to encourage flexion of the head and trunk and assist or resist the individual movements as necessary.

Action of the patient

To bring the buttocks forwards in the chair

1. Extend the right wrist and flex the forearm under the right armrest.

2. Using the right arm pull the trunk a little to the right and insert the left wrist behind the left hip. If wrist extension is strong, the forearm is pronated, if it is weak, the forearm is supinated (Fig. 11.3a).

3. Push on the right elbow on the back of the armrest. Flex the left elbow and push the left hip forwards and at the same time extend the head and lean backwards. The cushion will slide forward with the leg (Fig. 11.3b). Repeat to bring the right hip forwards. Figure 11.3c shows an alternative method for bringing the hips forward by pushing with both hands behind the hips at the same time. Two further methods are given in Chapter 10 page 112.

To lean forward over the legs place both hands on the rear wheels and at the same time flex the head, protract the shoulders and thrust forwards on the hands (Fig. 11.3d).

To lift the legs onto the plinth

1. To maintain balance hook the right forearm round the right chair handle.

2. Put the left wrist under the right knee and lift the leg by flexing the elbow (Fig. 11.3e). Pull the knee up to the chest by pulling the trunk upright with the right arm and leaning back in the chair.

3. Rest the left wrist on the right armrest and bring the right arm forwards onto the plinth (Fig. 11.3f).

4. Change the position of the arms so that the right wrist holds the knee, with the forearm supported on the armrest. The supinated left forearm moves down to support the lower leg (Fig. 11.3g).

5. Push the heel onto the plinth. Remove the right armrest as described on page 109.

6. Lift the left knee as for the right and hold the hip and knee in as much flexion as possible.

7. Maintain balance on the left elbow lift the lower leg with the right wrist (Fig. 11.3h).

8. Lean over to the right and cross the left leg over the right (Fig. 11.3i).

To transfer the trunk onto the plinth

The basic technique for this activity is the same as for lifting sideways on the mat.

1. Place the right hand on the plinth level with the upper thigh and the left hand on the cushion (Fig. 11.3j) or on the armrest where possible.

2. With the head and trunk flexed lift *upwards* and then to the right (Fig. 11.3k).

3. Several lifts will be necessary to complete the transfer (Fig. 11.3l).

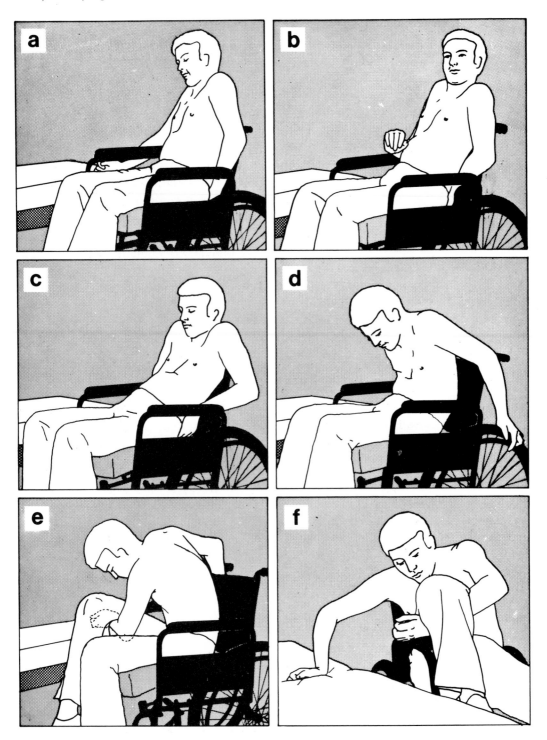

Fig. 11.3 Transferring to a plinth. Patient with a complete lesion below C$_6$ without triceps.

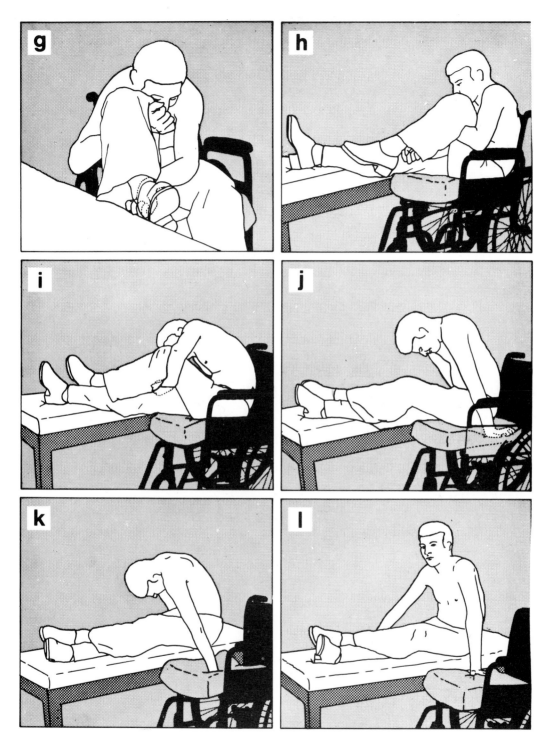

Fig. 11.3 (contd)

Removal of the footplates

The footplates need to be removed for most transfers.

To remove the right footplate

To transfer the right foot to the left footplate or to the floor:

1. Balance is maintained with the left hand on the armrest if the patient has a lesion at C_7, or with the left elbow or wrist hooked round the left chair handle if triceps is paralysed.

2. With the right wrist extended under the lower leg (Fig. 11.4a) flex the elbow and lift the foot over to the left footplate (Fig. 11.4b).

To remove the footplate (Fig. 11.4c):

1. With the wrist extended, release the lever by pushing it forwards with the dorsum of the hand (Fig. 11.4d).

2. Swing back the footplate using extension of the wrist (Fig. 11.4e).

3. Lift the footplate off the bracket using the dorsum of the hand and wrist extension (Fig. 11.4f).

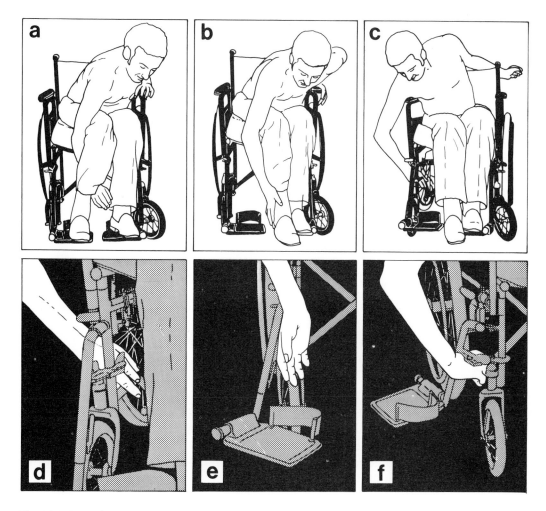

Fig. 11.4 Tetraplegic patient removing the footplate.

To transfer to the car (moving to the left)

Some patients with lesions at C_6 without triceps and those at C_7 with no hand function may find that a sliding board facilitates this transfer. The most useful dimensions of the sliding board have proved to be $24'' \times 7\frac{1}{2}'' \times 1\frac{1}{2}$ cm depth tapered at both ends. A notch at the end facilitates the handling of the board, and a loop may be necessary for some patients to enable them to remove the board after transfer.

Position of the chair

The chair is angled at approximately 30° to the side of the car. Remove both footplates or if preferred one only (the left in the example shown in Fig. 11.5).

Action of the patient

1. Lift the feet into the car as for transferring to the plinth. Remove the armrest.
2. Place a sliding board under the left thigh.
3. Lift using the left half of the sliding board and the right armrest or chair seat (Fig. 11.5a) keeping the head and trunk well flexed.
4. Repeat the lift as often as necessary, moving the hands a little to the left each time (Fig. 11.5b). The head and trunk must remain flexed with the nose almost touching the steering wheel during the later lifts (Fig. 11.5c).
5. Remove the sliding board from the right and adjust the legs in the sitting position (Fig. 11.5d).

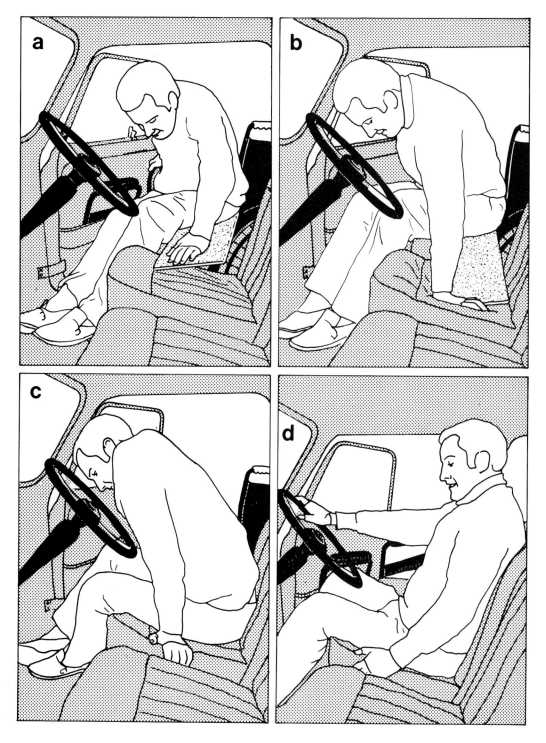

Fig. 11.5 Transferring to a car. Patient with a complete lesion below C_7 with wrist control only.

To transfer to the toilet (moving to the right)

Position of the chair

Place the chair at an angle of between 50° and 90° to the toilet seat. Many patients find the lift easier with the chair at right angles, because this position brings the armrest furthest from the toilet, closer to the handrail. Remove the footplates.

Position of the therapist

The therapist stands in front of the patient bracing his knees and feet and holding under the buttocks or in the trouser band. As the patient's proficiency increases, the therapist gradually withdraws her support.

Action of the patient

1. Check the position of the feet to see that they are flat on the floor and vertically beneath the knees so that the weight is over them. Remove the right armrest.
2. Keep the head and shoulders *flexed* throughout the transfer.
3. With the left hand on the armrest and the right on the rail, lift to the right (Fig. 11.6a and b).
4. With the left hand on the wheel and the right hand on the rail, lift further back onto the toilet (Fig 11.6c). To transfer back to the chair reverse the procedure.

In the absence of a wall rail, the experienced paraplegic patient can lift with his right hand on the toilet seat.

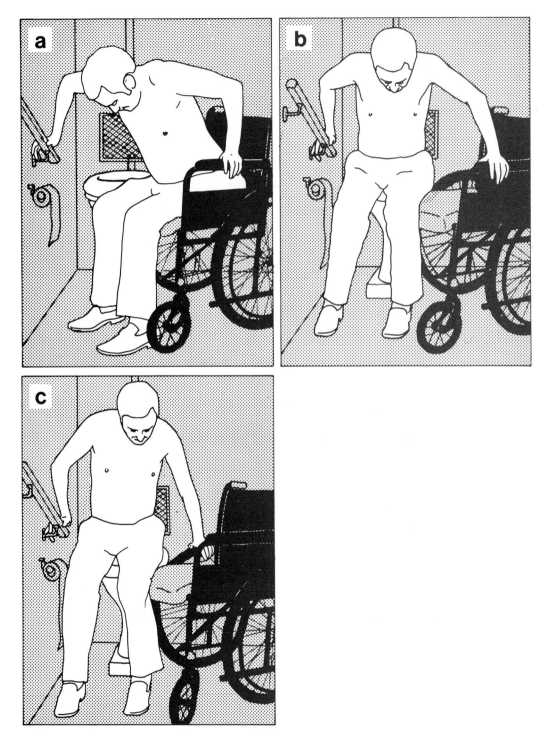

Fig. 11.6 Transferring to a toilet. Patient with a complete lesion below C$_7$ with wrist control only (note back support on toilet).

To transfer to the toilet through the back of the chair

This method can be used when spasticity is severe. For example, the patient may be at risk transferring sideways when there is a combination of hip extension and knee flexion spasticity.

The normal backrest can be replaced by one which opens throughout its length by means of a zipper. The patient lifts backwards as shown in Figure 11.7 with one hand on the rail and the other on the toilet seat. Relaxation of the extensor spasticity may be obtained by flexing one or both legs before lifting backwards.

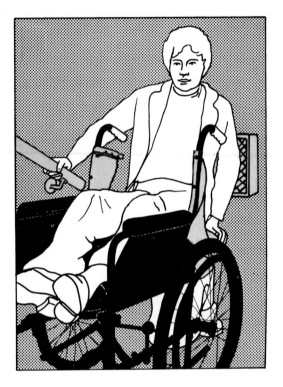

Fig. 11.7 Backwards transfer.

To transfer into an easy chair

This transfer is basically the same as the sideways transfer to the toilet, the arm of the easy chair being used instead of the wall rail. The wheelchair is positioned at right angles to the easy chair with the front edge of the seat approximately half way along the seat of the easy chair. This position brings the two lifting points closer together.

To transfer to the bath

The bath is filled with water before entering and drained before leaving. Bath transfer can be accomplished by patients with lesions at C_7 and below.

To transfer over the bath end

Action of the patient

1. Position the chair so that the feet almost touch the bath.
2. Lift both legs onto the edge of the bath (Fig. 11.8a).
3. Swing away the footplates (Fig. 118b).
4. Wheel forwards until the chair is adjacent to the bath (Fig. 11.8c).
5. Lift the buttocks forwards in the chair.
6. Continue lifting forwards with the right arm on the bath edge and the left arm on the armrest (Fig. 11.8d).
7. Transfer the left hand to the bath and lift onto the edge of the bath with the trunk almost fully flexed (Fig. 11.8e).
8. Maintaining the flexion, move the hands along the bath sides, lift and lower the body into the bath as gently as possible (Fig. 11.8f and g).

To get out of the bath reverse the procedure, flexing the legs before commencing to lift.

Those patients who are unable to lift the depth of the bath can use a low wooden bath seat as an interim step. The edge of the seat must be padded and care taken to ensure that the skin is not damaged during the lift.

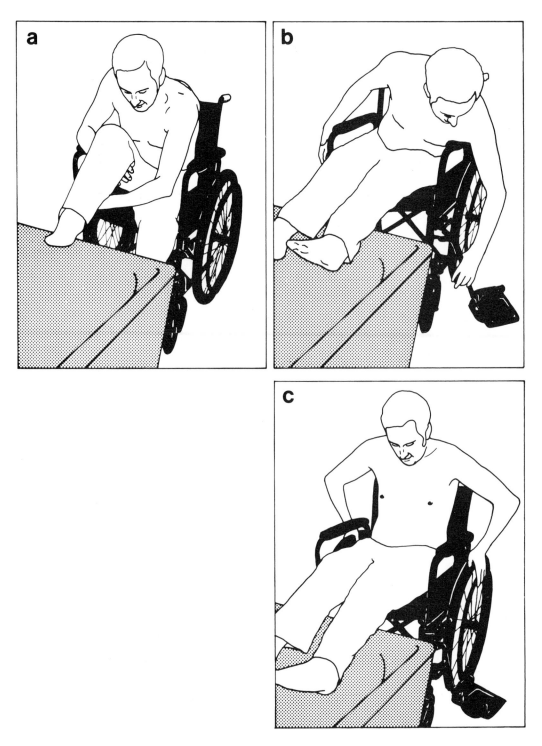

Fig. 11.8 Transfer over the bath end. Patient with a complete lesion below C₇ with wrist control only.

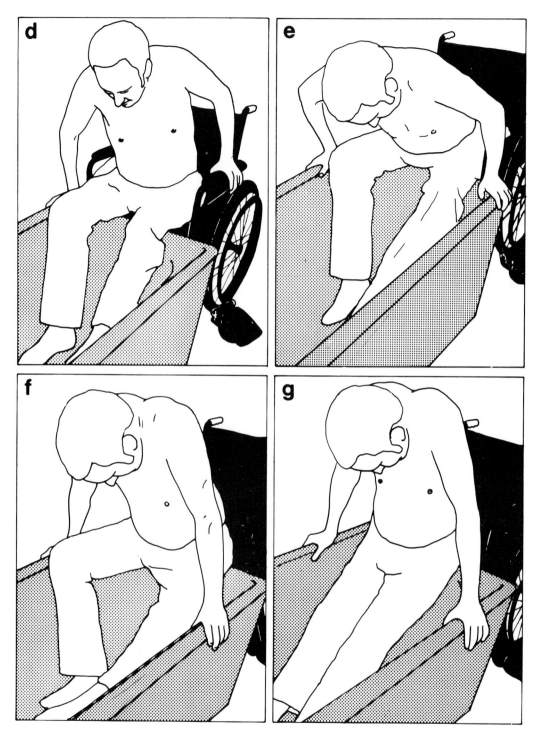

Fig. 11.8 (contd)

To transfer over the bath side

Position the chair sideways at an angle of 30° to the bath or facing the bath.

1. Lift the legs into the bath.
2. Lift onto the bath edge.
3. With one hand on each side of the bath, turn to face the bath end (Fig. 11.9).
4. Lift and lower gently into the bath.

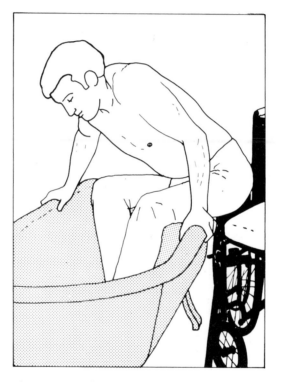

Fig. 11.9 Transfer over the bath side. Patient with a complete lesion below C_8.

Where there is a ledge behind the bath a combination of these two methods can be used. First transfer over the side onto the ledge, where the patient is more stable, and from there into the bath, as in Figure 11.8.

To transfer to the floor
The therapist

The therapist stands in front of the patient correcting his position and assisting him to maintain balance as necessary.

Action of the patient

    1. Remove the armrests.

    2. Lift with the left elbow on the backrest and the right hand on the wheel and pull the cushion out with the left hand (Fig. 11.10a).

    3. Remove the footplates and place the cushion between the front wheels for protection when sitting on the floor (Fig. 11.10b).

    4. Gripping the front of the seat supports lift the trunk (Fig. 11.10c) and allow the buttocks to slip forwards over the edge of the chair (Fig. 11.10d).

    5. Gradually lower the weight to the floor (Fig 11.10e).

Patients without abdominal muscles will need to extend the head and shoulders to tip the buttocks forwards off the chair at step 4. The extension is maintained to prevent the patient pitching forwards whilst lowering the trunk.

To lift back into the chair

Sitting with the back to the chair:

    1. Either place both hands on the front of the seat supports, or replace one footplate and place one hand on the top of the footplate fitting.

    2. Lift strongly, extending the head and neck (Fig. 11.10f).

    3. Contract the abdominals, if present, and depress the shoulders to pull the pelvis back onto the seat (Fig. 11.10g).

    4. Lift the feet onto the footplates.

To replace the cushion

Double the cushion and place it between the wheel and the hip (Fig. 11.10h). Lift on both wheels and the cushion 'springs' into place under the buttocks (Fig. 11.10i).

Alternative method for patients without abdominals

Replace the armrests. Double the cushion and place it low down between the back and the backrest. Lift on both armrests and the cushion 'springs' into position.

In both cases the position of the cushion may need final adjustment.

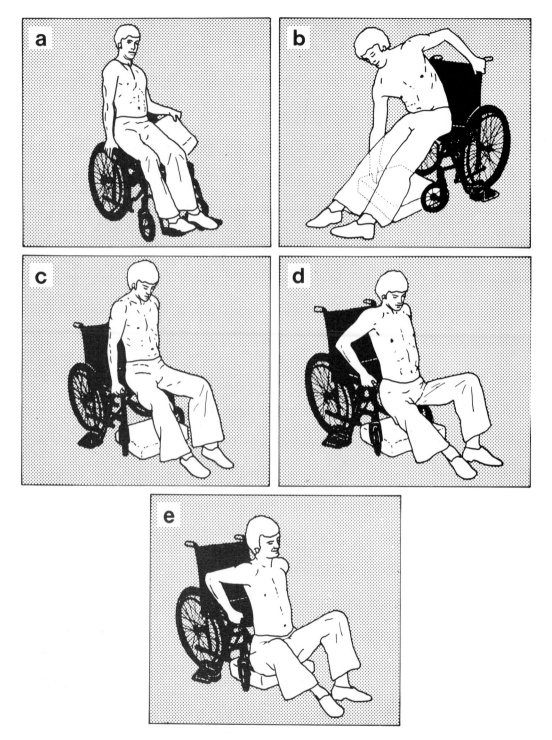

Fig. 11.10 Transfer to the floor. Patient with a complete lesion below T$_{11}$.

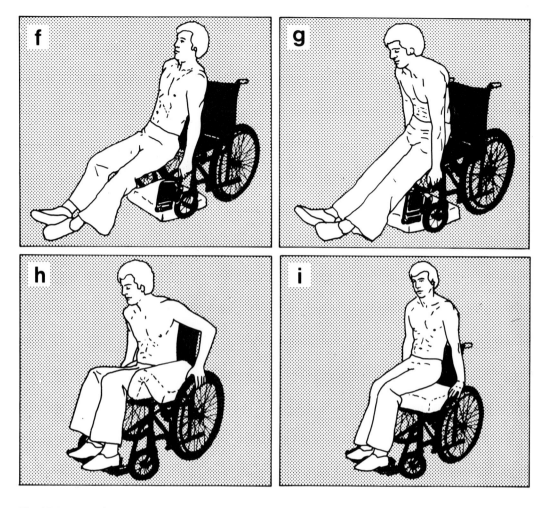

Fig. 11.10 (contd)

To transfer forwards onto the bed

The forwards transfer may be useful for the very young or for those who are overweight or severely spastic.

1. Lift the feet onto the bed.
2. Wheel the chair forwards until it is touching the bed.
3. Keeping the head and trunk flexed, lift forwards in the chair. Small children who cannot lift on the armrests push on the cushion (Fig. 11.11a). Repeated lifts may be necessary (Fig. 11.11b).
4. With the left hand on the bed and the right hand on the cushion lift the buttocks sideways onto the bed (Fig. 11.11c and d). Repeated lifts will be necessary.

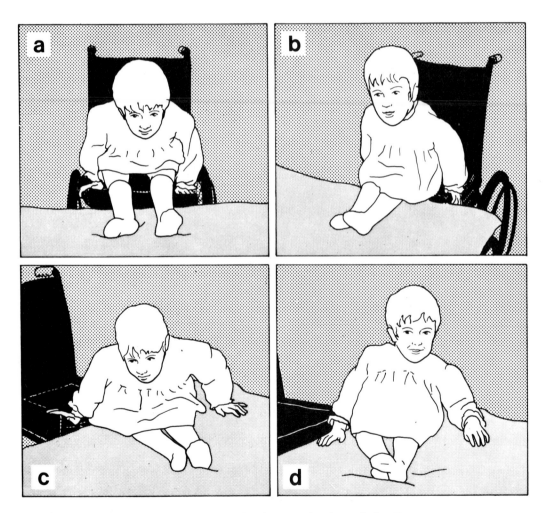

Fig. 11.11 Forwards transfer to the bed. Child with a complete lesion below T_{10}.

12

Gait training

All patients are encouraged to stand, and to walk where possible. Standing is considered important for the following reasons:

1. To prevent contractures developing in the lower limbs.
2. To minimise the development of osteoporosis of the long bones and thereby reduce the danger of recurrent fractures.
3. To stimulate the circulation.
4. To reduce spasticity.
5. To aid renal function.

The following is a general description of the capabilities of patients with varying lesions:

Patients with lesions at C_2–C_4:   Stand on the tilt table.
Patients with lesions at C_5–C_7:   Stand in bars.
Patients with lesions at C_6–T_5:   Walk in bars.
Patients with lesions at T_6–T_9:   Walk on crutches.
Patients with lesions at T_{10} and below: Achieve a functional gait.

The list is rudimentary and provides a guideline only, as patients will continually cross from one group to another in spite of their lesion. Some patients with lesions at T_6 use crutches for 80% of the day's activities whilst others at T_{12} walk only in bars or use a standing frame. As in all rehabilitation so much depends upon the physical proportions, age, sex, and previous medical history of the patient and even more upon his motivation.

Functional gait

The aim is to teach the use of both wheelchair and crutches so that the patient is equipped to use either as occasion demands. A widely increased sphere of independence is gained through crutch walking. Independent entrance can be obtained, for example, to buildings with small doorways, hotel accommodation, aircraft and trains. For the active patients the benefits gained in everyday life far outweigh the patience and effort involved in training.

Concern is sometimes expressed about the effect that weight bearing has on the shoulder joint. Research to determine the effect of the swing-through crutch walking gait on shoulder degeneration showed that no degenerative changes occurred, and there was an increase in the forearm bone density (Wing, 1983).

Appliances

From both the patient's and the medical point of view the appliances used to enable patients to stand are reduced to the minimum, and the patient is encouraged to put on his own appliances as soon as possible. The basic requirements are to fix the knee joints and to hold the feet in dorsiflexion. The overdevelopment of the trunk muscles, together with the creation of a new postural sense, render a pelvic band or spinal brace unnecessary for the great majority of patients. These appliances are prescribed for special cases. A full spinal brace is usually prescribed for children and also for young adults with a tendency to scoliosis. An abdominal belt may be helpful for patients with viseroptosis.

Calipers

Calipers, which allow the legs to bear the weight, are the only essential appliance for most patients. If standing is to minimise the formation of osteoporosis it is vital that the weight should go through the long bones. Ischial weight-bearing is to be avoided because of the danger of causing pressure sores. A bucket-type thigh corset is used. The knee supports need to be wide. They encircle the knee to prevent lateral movement and give adequate support to the paralysed joint (Fig. 12.1). Round sockets are used in the shoe with either back stops or toe raising springs. In a small number of cases with extreme plantar flexion spasticity, both may be needed. Ringlocks are commonly used, as the bar of the Hoffman joint does not fit easily under tight trousers.

The calipers are made of duralumin as they need to be as light as possible. Where patients are overweight or have severe spasticity, it may be necessary to replace the duralumin with steel. For patients with low lesions whose walking will be functional, ortholon cosmetic calipers may be prescribed. The lower section is moulded round the calf and heel and under the foot to just below the metatarso-phalangeal joints and the upper section round the back of the thigh.

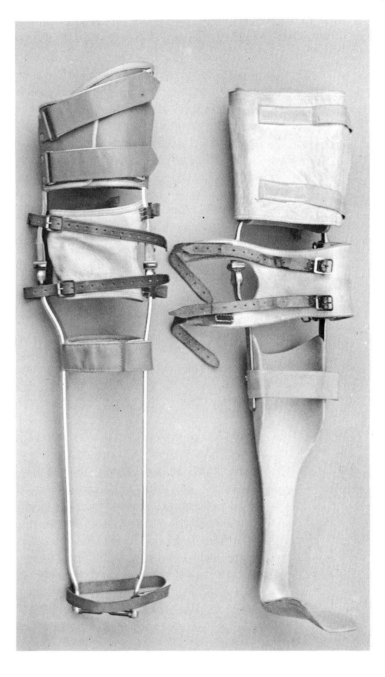

Fig. 12.1 Calipers.

These calipers are cosmetically more acceptable, but care must be taken to ensure that they do not cause pressure sores.

Caution *These calipers are unsuitable for patients with severe spasticity or oedema of the feet and lower legs.*

Calipers are available which have adjustable locked ankle joints (Scott, 1980). The correct angle to gain maximum stability is found with the patient standing in the balanced position in the bars with hips hyperextended and feet dorsiflexed beyond 90° (see p. 154). The ankle joint is locked with the patient standing in this position. The shoe is flat to take a steel plate and is permanently fixed to the caliper which is made of steel and is heavier than if made from duralumin. As these calipers give greater stability they may be particularly useful for patients with lesions between T_6 and T_9 (Duffus, 1983).

Some therapists encourage and some discourage gait for patients with lesions as high as T_6. Calipers are expensive. Research has shown that the majority of paraplegic patients use their wheelschairs as their main means of locomotion, using calipers for standing and exercise only. Approximately 10% use calipers for functional activities and a little less than one-third never use them at all (Haln, 1970; Mickelberg, 1981). Predictive factors are needed to identify those patients who will become and remain functional walkers.

Plaster of Paris leg splints

Posterior shells of plaster of Paris are made for each patient and used to stabilise the knees until calipers are available. The shells extend from 2 inches below the ischial tuberosities to 2 inches above the malleolii. It may be necessary to reinforce the plasters with a strip of steel or Kramer wire for patients who are overweight or who have severe spasticity. Temporary toe raising springs are used with these splints to hold the foot in dorsiflexion. They consist of a webbing band round the leg, with adjustable straps, a short spring and a narrow webbing band under the shoe (Fig. 12.2).

Modular calipers can now be kept in stock to fit on a temporary basis in place of plaster of Paris leg splints. They appear to be of limited use and most physiotherapists prefer to make plaster splints.

Shoes

Shoes for use with calipers should provide good support for the feet, be made of soft leather and without toe caps. To prevent pressure sores all the inside seams, particularly around the heel, must be smooth. Leather soles stitched to the uppers provide the most suitable support for the sockets, back stops, D rings, or T straps if necessary. To accommodate for slight oedema and avoid damage when putting

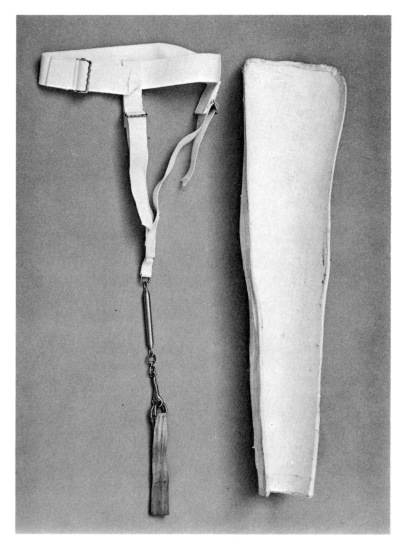

Fig. 12.2 Temporary toe-raising spring and plaster of Paris splint.

them on, the shoe fitting should be *at least* half a size larger than the size previously worn.

STANDING

Standing between parallel bars

Because of the loss of all postural and equilibrium reactions below the level of the lesion, a new postural sense must be developed in the erect position. Compensation by sight for the loss of sensation is essential, and a long mirror is used at the end of the bars. Patients without muscle control at the hips lift their legs by the action of latissimus dorsi and the associated action of trapezius and shoulder girdle muscles. Postural sense in standing is developed largely through the action of these 'bridge' muscles.

Position of the wheelchair

The chair is positioned with the supporting cross bar of the bars behind the front wheels, if possible. This will prevent the chair from slipping backwards.

Height of the bars

For the efficient use of latissimus dorsi and triceps the bars must be at the correct height. With the hand on the bar and the shoulders relaxed, the elbow must be slightly flexed. This usually brings the wrist approximately level with the great trochanter, but this depends upon individual physical proportions. For the initial stand the height of the bars is determined by guesswork. After seeing the patient on his feet the therapist must make the necessary adjustments. It is a common error to have the bars too high. In this case elevation of the shoulder renders depression almost impossible and the patient cannot lift the leg effectively. With the bars too low stability can be gained only when the patient leans forwards with his weight on his hands.

To stand a tetraplegic patient

Many patients have sufficient motor power to maintain their balance in standing and even to walk in bars, without having sufficient power to lift themselves into the standing position. Occasionally vasomotor disturbances occur on standing. If necessary an abdominal support or binder can be applied temporarily to help prevent pooling of the blood in the splanchnic vessels. Fainting is more likely to occur when the patient is tall and thin (Figoni, 1984).

Position of the patient

1. Lift forward in the chair until the heels touch the ground.
2. Place the arms round the therapist's neck.
3. Lean forward with the chin over the therapist's shoulder for extra support if necessary.

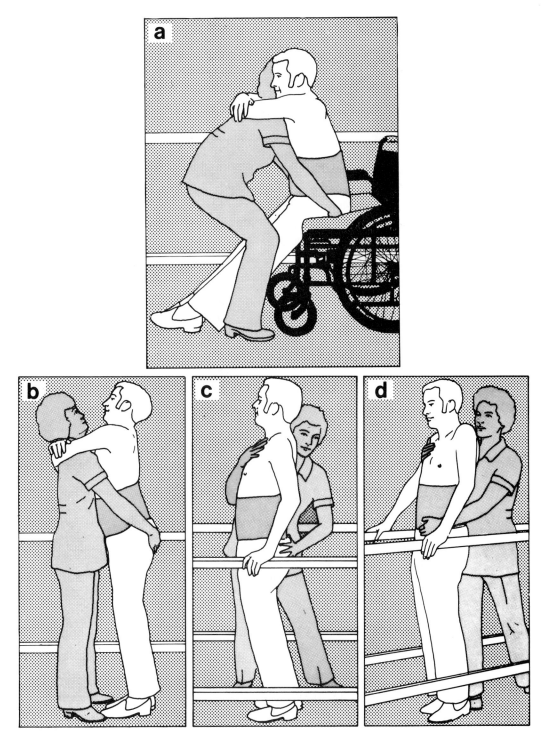

Fig. 12.3 Standing a patient with a cervical lesion (note abdominal belt).

The therapist

1. Stand astride the patient's legs.
2. Place the hands under the buttocks (Fig. 12.3a).
3. Turn the head to one side, e.g. the left so that the patient can get a good grip with his arms around the neck.
4. Brace the knees against the patient's legs and use them as a pivot point to pull the patient into standing.
5. As the patient becomes erect take a few steps backwards until his weight is over his feet (Fig. 12.3b).
6. Pull the buttocks forwards and encourage the patient to extend his head and shoulders. The patient with functional triceps can put his hands on the therapist's shoulders or on the bars and push his upper trunk into extension. When balance is obtained the patient puts his hands on the bars.

To get behind the patient

Keeping the hips in extension with the left hand and the upper trunk extended with the right arm, move behind the patient by passing under his right arm. At the same time slide the arms around the patient's trunk to maintain his position (Fig. 12.3c).

To balance the patient

Brace one hip against the patient's sacrum to maintain hyperextension of his hips. Prevent forward or lateral movement of the trunk with the right hand on the upper thorax and the left hand on the pelvis (Fig. 12.3d). Watching in the mirror the therapist helps the patient to find his point of balance and encourages him to hold it without her support. When this has been achieved resisted exercises can be given to improve balance and co-ordination. If a young and active patient with a lesion at C_7 or C_8 is anxious to walk, swing-to gait can be taught as for the paraplegic patient.

To stand a paraplegic patient

The therapist

Stand facing the patient, with the feet either side of the patient's legs, ready to grip with the knees to prevent the feet from sliding forwards.

Step-standing may be preferred, as in Figure 12.4a. Hold the patient under the buttocks and pull the hips forwards as the patient lifts.

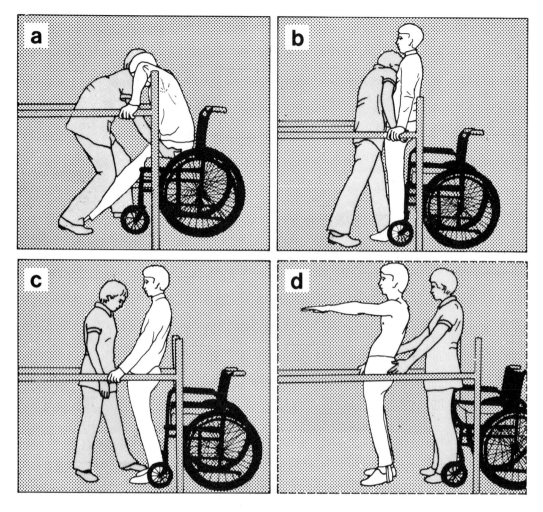

Fig. 12.4 (a–c) Standing a paraplegic patient. (d) Balance exercise in the bars. Patient with a complete lesion below T_5.

Action of the patient

1. Sitting well back in the chair, lean forward and place the hands at the end of the bars with the elbows vertically above the wrists (Fig. 12.4a). This position allows the patient to stand by *pushing down* on the bars. The tendency to reach along the bars and pull up, must be avoided.

2. Push down on the hands and stretch *upwards*, not forwards (Fig. 12.4b).

3. As the weight comes over the feet, hyperextend the hips and at the same time extend the head and retract the shoulders.

4. Move the hands a short distance forwards along the bars (Fig. 12.4c). If the patient is tall or overweight a second therapist may be needed to push the feet back as the patient lifts. This will reduce the effort required by the patient.

The therapist moves behind the patient giving support as already described.

Posture correction

The standing posture is corrected so that:

1. Weight goes through the heels.

2. Legs are inclined only a few degrees forwards of 90° at the ankle.

3. Hips are slightly extended so that the line of gravity lies behind the hip joints through the knee joints and slightly in front of the ankle joints to prevent the 'jack-knife' fall forwards.

4. Spine is as upright as possible. Some adjustment must be made in the upper thoracic spine to compensate for the hyperextended hips. Overcorrection must be avoided.

5. Bars are held with the hands approximately level with the toes.

6. Shoulders are relaxed.

The posture of the patient with useful abdominal muscles should be almost erect except for the slight hyperextension necessary at the hip joints. As the level of the lesion rises a greater degree of compensation will be necessary at the hip joints. In all cases *overcorrection* should be avoided. If the patient is allowed to lean forward with the weight over the toes and with the spine and shoulders extended, he will be unable to lift the weight off his feet. A second mirror placed at the side of the patient may assist him to correct his posture by showing the anteroposterior deviations from the vertical.

There is a fine point between over- and under-correction. This position provides the basic balance point from which all gait training proceeds.

Duration of the stand

Depending upon the height of the lesion the patient may remain on his feet for only 2 minutes or up to five or 10 minutes on the first day. A *gradual* increase in the duration of the stand is most important in order to allow the circulation to adapt with the minimum ill effect on the patient.

Initially it is more beneficial to stand two or three times for a few moments only than to stand once for a longer period. The constant change in posture stimulates the vascular system and promotes a more rapid establishment of vasomotor adjustment.

To sit down

The therapist, holding the patient under the buttocks and controlling his legs with her knees and feet, allows him to sit down gradually.

Action of the patient

With the feet approximately a foot's length from the chair:

1. Hyperextend the hips and place the hands in their original position on the bars.
2. Take the weight on the arms.
3. Flex the head and trunk and lower the weight gently until the bottocks reach the chair.

Caution *Care must be taken to ensure that the patient does not knock his hips against the sides of the chair, or drop his weight suddenly onto the buttocks. Bruising, both superficial and in the deeper tissues, can easily occur.*

When resting in the chair, with splints or calipers on the legs, the heels must be supported on a stool; otherwise the weight of the leg is taken on the upper end of the femur. If preferred calipers can be unlocked at the knee joints.

Exercises in standing

As control is gained over the upper thorax, the therapist can place both hands around the hips to support only the pelvis. The hands are placed along the iliac crest, with the fingers over the anterior, superior iliac spine. With the hands in this position, the therapist can pull the pelvis back with her fingers (Fig. 12.5a) push it forwards with the heel of her hand (Fig. 12.5b) give pressure downwards or lift upwards (Fig. 12.5c). In this way the therapist has complete control of the patient and can assist or resist movement in any direction.

Balance exercises

Watching his position in the mirror, the patient is taught to:

1. Hold, move out of and regain the correct posture.
2. Maintain balance whilst lifting one hand off the bar (Fig. 12.4d). Progression is made by moving the arm in all directions, and later, to repeating this with the eyes closed.
3. Move both hands forwards and backwards along the bars.

Exercises for strength and control

Before commencing gait training the patient must learn to tilt his pelvis by using latissimus dorsi and to become aware of the degree of control he can achieve with this compensatory mechanism.

Pelvic side tilting

To 'hitch' the left leg:
   Place the left hand on the bar only slightly in front of the left hip, and the right hand about half a foot length further forwards. Keeping the elbow straight press firmly down on the left hand and *depress the shoulder*.
   The leg must be lifted *upwards* and not forwards.

To lift both feet off the ground and control the pelvis

Place both hands on the bars slightly in front of the hip joints. Push down on the bars, with the elbows straight, and depress the shoulders. To gain control of the pelvis, the patient should practise holding himself at full and at part lift, rotating the trunk and tilting the pelvis with the feet lifted off the ground.

Resisted trunk exercises

For greater efficiency in balance, strength and control, resisted trunk exercises in the standing and 'lifting' positions and resisted 'hitching' are also given.

Passive stretch in standing

Where strong spasm in the hip flexors and abdominal muscles prevents the patient from assuming the erect posture, a passive stretch can be given. The therapist gives firm pressure forwards with her hip against the patient's sacrum, and with her hands pulls backwards over the front of the shoulder joints.

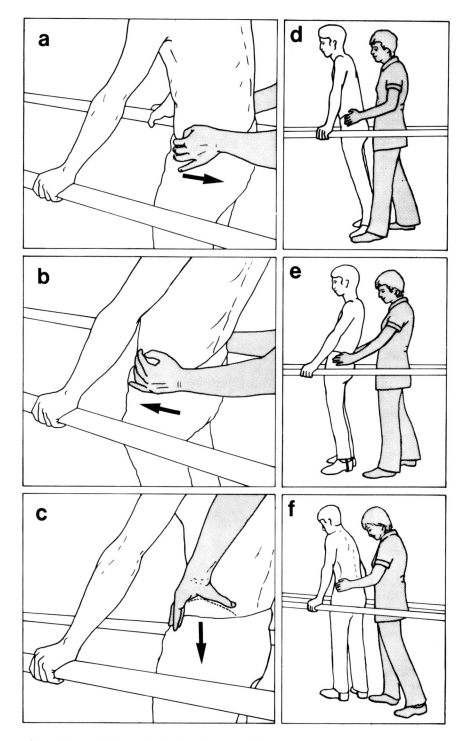

Fig. 12.5 (a–c) Position of the therapist's hands. (d & e) Swing-to gait. (f) Four-point gait.

If the position is maintained for a few moments the spasticity usually relaxes and the patient is able to maintain his balance.

Caution 1. *Stretching must always be performed with extreme care. Unskilled passive stretching has resulted in fracture of the neck of the femur. The top of the caliper becomes the fulcrum and the strain is transferred to the femoral neck.*

2. Until the spasm relaxes the patient may experience some difficulty in breathing. The spasticity is initially increased by the stretch, and the tightness of the abdominal muscles may prevent adequate movement of the diaphragm.

3. The therapist must make sure that she has no hard objects in her pocket which could cause pressure.

Standing frames

Where walking is impractical, a standing frame may be used once balance in the bars is achieved. The Oswestry frame and the Godfrey Standing Aid are both useful examples. With additional straps the former can be used by tetraplegic as well as paraplegic patients.

GAIT

There are three types of gait used:

1. Swing-to- gait
2. Four-point gait
3. Swing-through gait.

Controlled walking is achieved only through perseverance, perfect timing, rhythm and co-ordination.

The patient is taught always:

1. To move the hands first.
2. To walk slowly and place his feet accurately.
3. To take the weight through the feet and so ensure that the hands can relax between each step.
4. To lift the body *upwards* and not to drag the legs forwards.

An accurate technique must be achieved in bars if crutch walking is to be successful.

Where it is anticipated that the patient will become an accomplished walker, it is usual to commence training with the four-point gait. It is easier to learn to use the latissimus dorsi muscles at first separately and then together than vice versa.

GAIT TRAINING IN THE BARS

Swing-to gait

This is the universal gait because it is both the simplest and the safest. All patients with lesions above T_{10} are normally taught this gait first.

The therapist

The therapist stands behind the patient with her hands over the iliac crests. Assistance is given to lift, to control the tilt of the pelvis and to transfer weight as necessary.

Action of the patient

1. Balance in the hyperextended position.
2. Move the hands, either separately or together, forwards along the bars approximately half-a-foot length in front of the toes.
3. Lean forward, with the head and shoulders over the hands (Fig. 12.5d), and *lift* the legs, which will swing forward to follow the position of the head and shoulders. The step is short and the feet must drop just *behind* the level of the hands (Fig. 12.5e). To achieve this the lift must be released quickly, otherwise the feet will travel too far and land between or in front of the hands. When on crutches it is unstable and therefore dangerous to have the feet and hands in line. It must therefore be avoided in the bars. The swing-to gait is a 'staccato' gait with no follow through: 'lift and drop'.
   The patient should also be taught to swing backwards along the bars.

To turn in the bars

The turn is achieved in two movements by turning through 90° each time.
   To turn to the right:

1. Place the left hand forward about a foot length along the bars and the right hand either level with or a little behind the trunk.
2. Lift and twist the shoulders and upper trunk to the right. The feet land facing the bar to the right (Fig. 12.6a).
3. Balance in this position and move the left hand across to the right bar (Fig. 12.6b).
4. Twisting the upper trunk to the right, place the right hand on the opposite bar.
5. Lift the feet round to a central position between the bars (Fig. 12.6c).

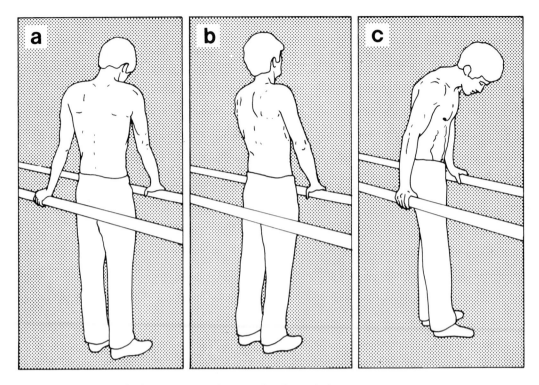

Fig. 12.6 Turning in the bars. Patient with a complete lesion below T_{11}.

Four-point gait

This gait is the slowest and most difficult and is only achieved on crutches by accomplished walkers. It facilitates turning and manoeuvring in confined spaces. It also provides an excellent training exercise in strength, balance and control.

The therapist

The therapist holds the pelvis in the usual way. Both by instruction and by correction with her hands, she emphasises each move, ensuring that the patient achieves it correctly. Only when the patient consistently makes a single movement correctly does the therapist stop correcting that component. The patient needs to see and 'feel' the correct posture at each move, and therefore constant repetition is necessary.

Action of the patient

To take a step forward with the left leg

1. Place the right hand forward about half-a-foot length along the bar and the left one just in front of the hip joint.

2. Take the weight on the right leg, so that the hip is *over* the right foot and the knee and ankle in a vertical line.

3. With the left shoulder slightly protracted push on the left hand and depress the shoulder (Fig. 12.5f). The effort is to 'lift' the leg *upwards*.

4. As the left leg is lifted it swings forward to follow the shoulder. The 'lift' is released when a large enough step has been made. (Small steps should be taken initially, but the foot must always land *in front of* the hand.)

5. Take the weight over the left leg.

6. Move the left hand forward along the bar in preparation for moving the right leg. Pelvic rotation must be avoided.

The following are possible reasons for an inadequate lift:

1. Some weight remains on the moving leg.
2. The hands are too far forward.
3. The weight may be over the toes and not back over the heels, in which case the *trunk* may be hyperextended and the legs consequently inclined too far forward.
4. Insufficient depression of the shoulder girdle on the side of the moving leg.
5. The bars are too high or too low.
6. The lift is not held for sufficient time to allow the leg to swing forward.

To take a step backward with the left leg

1. Place the left hand slightly behind the hip joint.
2. Lift the leg and at the same time lean forward on that side.
3. Bend the elbow and 'flip' the leg backwards.

Swing-through gait

This gait requires skilled balance, but it is the fastest and most useful.

The therapist

The therapist gives assistance where necessary with her hands controlling the pelvis until the patient can accurately and slowly perform the movements. The forward thrust of the pelvis to push the weight over the feet usually needs to be emphasised.

Action of the patient

1. Place the hands forwards along the bars as for the swing-to gait.

2. Lean forward and take the weight on the hands.

3. Push down on the bars, depress the shoulder girdle and lift both legs. The lift must be sustained until the legs have swung forwards to land the same distance in front of the hands as they were originally behind. Considerably more effort is required than for the swing-to gait.

4. As the weight is lifted and the legs swing forwards, hyperextend the hips, extend the head and *retract the shoulders*

5. To move the trunk forwards over the feet, push on the hands, extending the elbows and adducting the shoulders. When the weight is firmly on the feet move the hands along the bars for the next step.

GAIT TRAINING ON CRUTCHES

Progression is made to crutch walking only when the technique between the bars is good. The height of the elbow crutches is checked as for the bars.

The change from walking in bars to crutch walking is considerable, and all patients are initially unstable and fearful. A high degree of balance skill is essential and this is only achieved with perseverance and much practice.

Balance exercises

Balance on crutches is trained in the same way as when balancing in the bars (Fig. 12.7a). Resisted work is also given to enable the patient to gain adequate control over the trunk and pelvis.

Walking on crutches

Swing-to and four-point gaits are taught first, and progression is made to swing-through (Fig. 12.7b and c).

Until the new postural sense is established training is again carried out in front of a mirror.

Progression in the four-point gait may be made by using one bar and one crutch if preferred. Otherwise progression is directly onto two crutches, as there is less tendency to trunk and pelvic rotation.

The technique for each gait is the same as already described for walking in bars. Much greater skill is required and several weeks of practice will be needed to acquire the necessary balance and co-ordination.

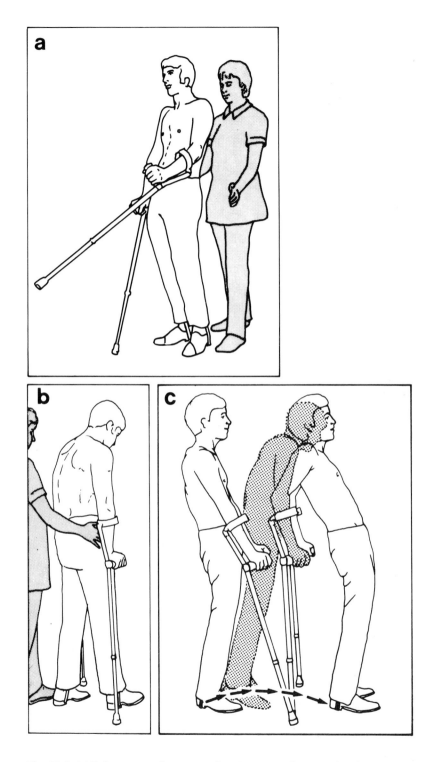

Fig. 12.7 (a) Balance exercise on crutches. Patient with a complete lesion below T_5.
(b) Four-point gait. (c) Swing-through gait. Patient with a complete lesion below T_{12}.

To transfer from chair to crutches

An unaided exit from a chair is essential if crutch walking is to be functional. There are three techniques used to get into and out of the chair with crutches:

1. Forwards technique
2. Sideways technique
3. Backwards technique.

All three methods are taught where possible, and the patient chooses that which he finds easiest.

Forwards technique

Severe abdominal and/or flexor spasticity which prohibits the necessary hyperextension at the hips, or excessive height may prevent a patient accomplishing this technique. When the patient is well over average height with the extra length primarily in the legs, the elbows are higher than the shoulders with the crutches in position for the lift. Latissimus dorsi and triceps are thus at a mechanical disadvantage and a balanced lift is impossible.

The therapist

The therapist stands in front of the patient astride the legs and ready to give support with her hands around the scapula region (Fig. 12.8).

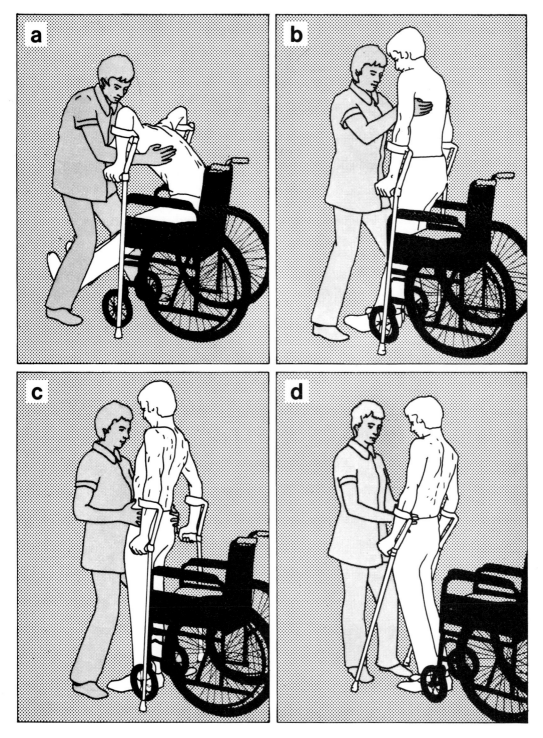

Fig. 12.8 Chair to crutches—forwards technique. Patient with a complete lesion below T_6.

Action of the patient

1. Check the position of the chair and swing away the footplates. During early training, when the weight distribution may be incorrect a feeling of stability is given if the chair is backed against a wall.

2. Sit well back in the chair (Fig. 12.9a).

3. Place the crutches midway between the front and rear wheels, level with each other and equidistant from the sides of the chair (Fig. 12.9b). To avoid rotation during the lift the position of the crutches must be accurate.

4. Lean forward over the crutches and balance.

5. Lift on the crutches, adducting and extending the shoulders.

6. The feet are lifted backwards, and as the weight goes onto them, hyperextend the hips and retract the shoulders (Fig. 12.9c).

7. When balanced move the crutches forward and assume the correct standing position (Fig. 12.9d).

To sit down reverse the procedure, as in Figures 12.9d–a

If the physical proportions of the patient are suitable, an alternative method is shown in Figure 12.9e. The short patient reaches back with his hands, releases the crutch handles and grasps the armrests. Such patients may be able to stand up in the same way. To prevent trauma, which could result in haemorrhage and bursa formation, sitting down should be done slowly without bumping on the chair.

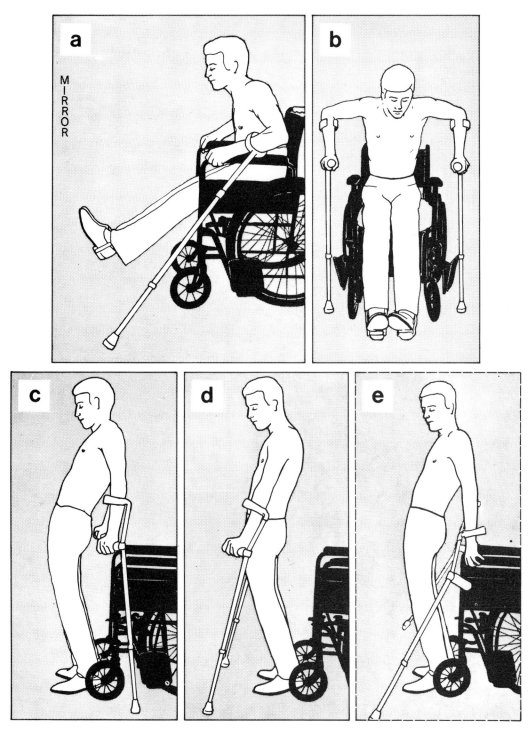

Fig. 12.9 (a–d) Chair to crutches — forwards technique. Patient with a complete lesion below T_9. (e) Short patient sitting down.

Sideways technique

Some patients of under-average height are able to get out of the chair using one crutch and an armrest:

1. Put the left arm through the forearm support, position the left crutch and grasp the armrest.
2. Turn through 45° towards the left armrest.
3. Place the right crutch in front and to the left of the mid-line of the chair.
4. Lift on both arms (Fig. 12.10a and b).
5. With the weight on the feet, balance on the right crutch and grasp the left crutch handle.

Reverse the procedure to sit down.

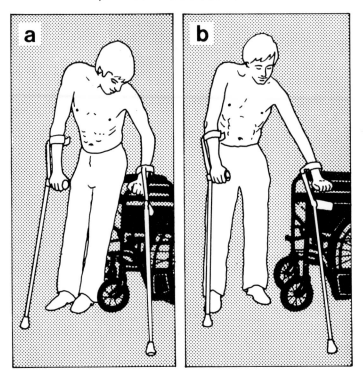

Fig. 12.10 Chair to crutches — sideways technique.

Backwards technique

The therapist stands in front of the patient ready to control the pelvis or legs as necessary.

To turn to the left:

Action of the patient (see pp. 170–171)

1. Cross the right leg over the left (Fig. 12.11a).
2. Lift the buttocks to the right side of the chair (Fig. 12.11b).
3. Turn the trunk to the left moving the left hand to the right armrest and the right hand to the left armrest (Fig. 12.11c).
4. Push on both armrests to stand (Fig. 12.11d) facing the chair.
5. Hitch the feet to the left (Fig. 12.11e).
6. Put each hand through the crutch forearm rest and return to holding the armrest (Fig. 12.11f).
7. Grasp the handgrips in turn.
8. Walk backwards away from the chair (Fig. 12.11g).

Reverse the procedure to sit down.

Stairs

Climbing stairs is normally functional for patients with good abdominal muscles. Some young and active patients with lesions between T_6 and T_{10}, with or without a spinal brace, may also become efficient and independent.

Patients can climb the stairs either forwards or backwards. The forwards technique is usually taught first because it has the advantage that the patient can see where he is going. Most agile patients with good abdominal muscles will learn both methods and make their own choice. Where there is severe abdominal and/or hip flexor spasticity the degree of hyperextension easily obtainable at the hip joints may be too limited for the forwards technique.

Two rails are used initially, progression being made to one rail and one crutch. Finally, the second crutch must be carried, usually in the crutch hand, as illustrated (Fig. 12.12).

The therapist

The therapist always stands behind the patient. She holds the trouser band with one hand and grasps the patient round the waist with the other. After the initial attempts both hands can be placed around the pelvis in the usual position and assistance given, as necessary, until the technique is mastered.

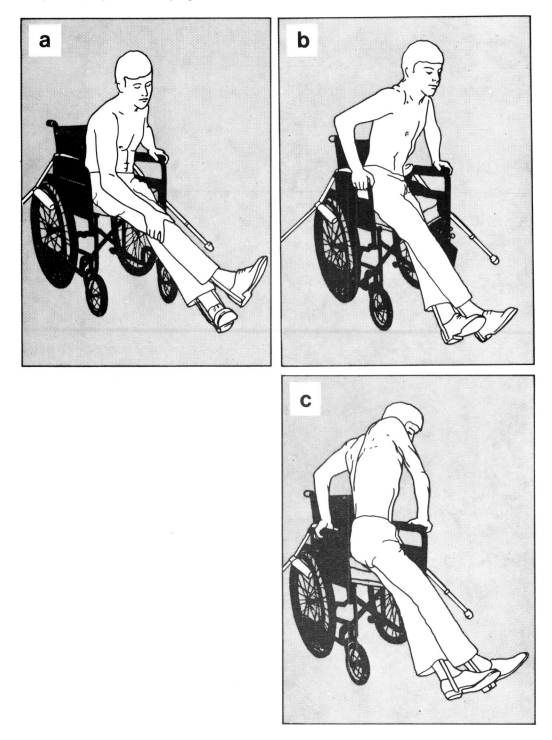

Fig. 12.11 Chair to crutches — backwards technique. Patient with a complete lesion below T_{12}.

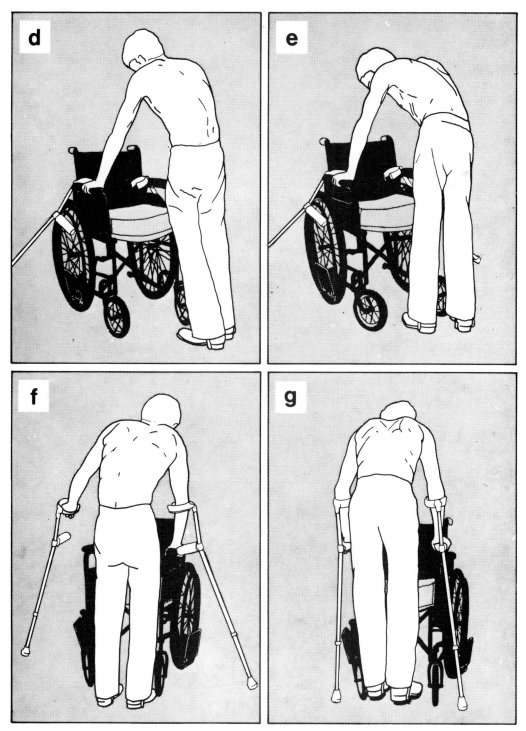

Fig. 12.11 (contd)

Forwards technique using one rail and one crutch

To walk upstairs

1. Standing close to the rail, grasp it approximately half-a-foot length in front of the toes.
2. Place the right crutch on the stair above and level with the hand on the rail (Fig. 12.12a). The hands must be level to avoid trunk rotation when lifting. The tendency to grasp the rail too far forwards and 'pull' must be avoided.
3. Lean over the hands and lift as high as possible, keeping the trunk and pelvis in the horizontal plane (Fig. 12.12b).
4. As soon as the feet land on the stair above, hyperextend the hips to find the balance point (Fig. 12.12c).

To walk downstairs

1. Standing close to the rail and keeping the body in the horizontal plane, place the right crutch close to the edge of the same stair.
2. Place the left hand down the rail on a level with the crutch (Fig. 12.12d).
3. Lift and swing the feet down to the stair below (Fig. 12.12e).
4. Hyperextend the hips and retract the shoulders as soon as the feet touch the ground (Fig. 12.12f).

Very short patients may need to put the crutch on the stair below the feet and lift down to the crutch.

Backwards technique using one rail and one crutch

To walk upstairs

1. Balance in hyperextension whilst placing the left hand higher up the rail and the crutch on the stair above, keeping the hands level (Fig. 12.12f).
2. Lift backwards (Fig. 12.12e).
3. Regain the balance (Fig. 12.12d).

To walk downstairs

1. Place the crutch on the edge of the same stair as the feet, with the hands level (Fig. 12.12c).
2. Lift the feet backwards to the edge of the stair.
3. Lean forwards on the hands, lift and 'flick' the pelvis backwards (Fig. 12.12b).
4. Drop the feet onto the stair below (Fig. 12.12a).

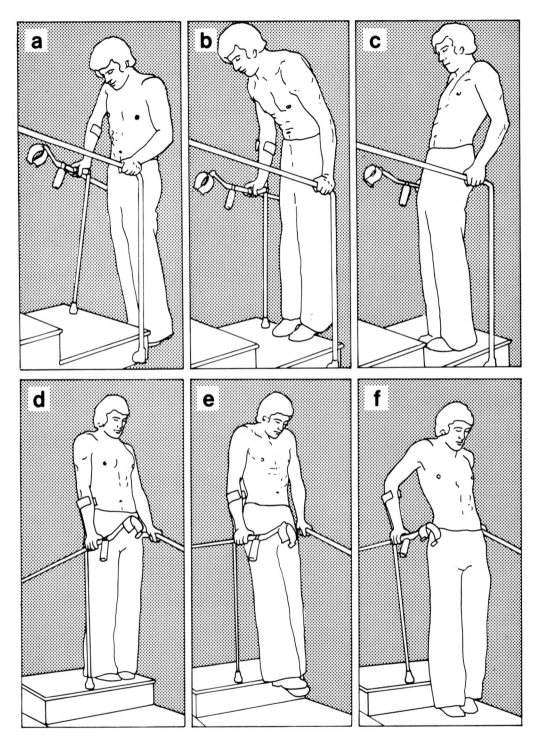

Fig. 12.12 Climbing and descending stairs. Patient with a complete lesion below T$_{11}$.

Kerbs

Kerbs are negotiated by putting the crutches on the kerb first and then taking a swing-through step onto the pavement. The same technique is used to descend a kerb. A long shallow step can be mounted in the same way.

Patients are not taught to ascend flights of narrow steps on two crutches.

To get out of a car onto crutches

1. Turn to face the open door and lift the legs out of the car.
2. Lock the knee joints.
3. With the window open, use the window-ledge and the back of the seat, or the seat and a crutch to lift into standing.
4. Balance with the hips hyperextended and take hold of each crutch in turn.

To get down and up from the floor onto crutches

Crutches to floor

The therapist stands behind the patient and controls the pelvis, feet and legs, as necessary.

1. From the standing position on the mat (Fig. 12.13a) 'walk' the crutches forward one by one (Fig. 12.13b) until the hips and trunk are sufficiently flexed for the outstretched hand to reach the floor.

2. Balance on the right crutch, release the left crutch and put the left hand on the floor (Fig. 12.13c).

3. Balance on the left hand, release the right crutch and put the right hand on the floor (Fig. 12.13d).

4. 'Walk' forward on the hands until lying prone (Fig. 12.13e).

Floor to crutches

The therapist may need to assist the patient to get the weight over his feet initially.

1. In prone-lying make sure the ankles and toes are dorsiflexed so that the feet are vertical (Fig. 12.13f).

2. Position the crutches, tips forward, well in front of the body and put both forearms through the forearm supports.

3. Press up on the hands, and at the same time use the abdominal muscles to pull the pelvis towards the hands and so prevent the legs being pushed backwards.

4. Maintaining the action of the abdominal muscles, 'walk' the hands towards the feet, trailing the crutches (Fig. 12.13g) *until the weight is over the feet* (Fig. 12.13h).

5. Balance on the left hand, grasp the right crutch handle and place the crutch on the floor (Fig. 12.13i).

6. Balance on the right crutch and take hold of the left crutch in a similar manner. Balance on both crutches (Fig. 12.13j).

7. 'Walk' the crutches towards the feet until standing erect (Fig. 12.13k).

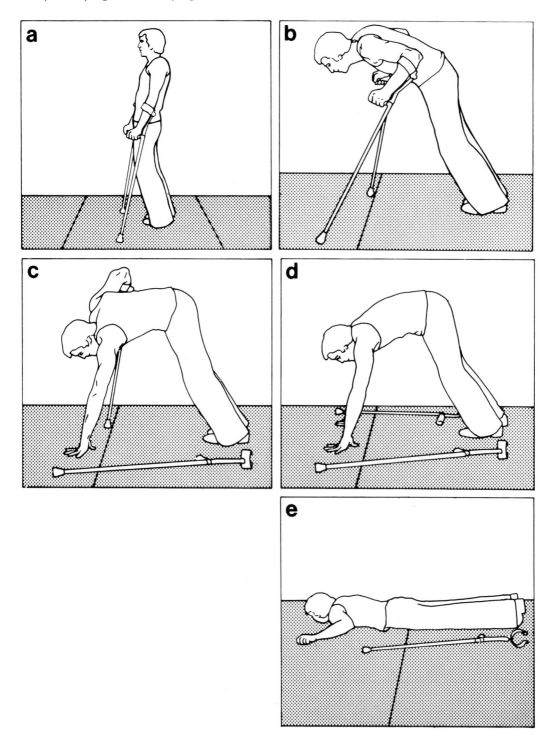

Fig. 12.13 Crutches to floor. Patient with a complete lesion below T$_{11}$.

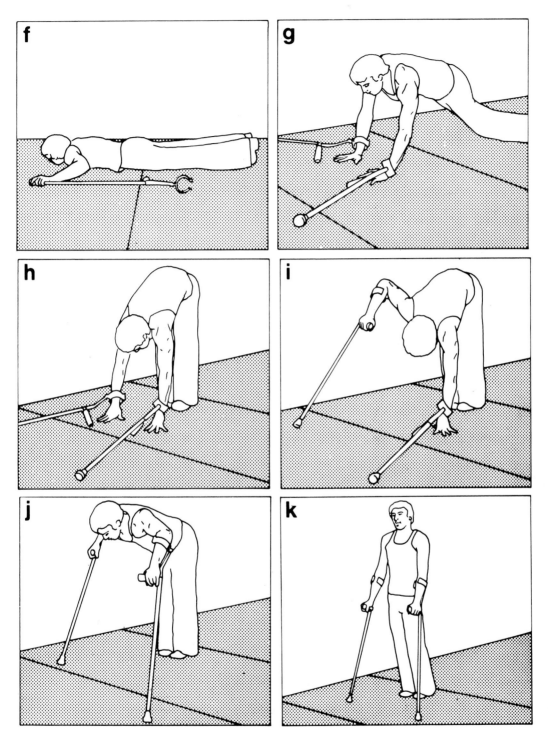

Fig. 12.13 (contd)

Final functional activities on crutches

The patient is taught to walk on slopes and over uneven ground such as grass and shale. He must also learn to open and close a door, to sit in and rise from an easy chair and to sit down and rise from table by pushing down on the table with one hand and using the crutch in the other.

13

The ultra-high lesion

Injuries to the upper cervical spine C_1–C_3 paralyse the diaphragm as well as the other muscles of respiration and prove fatal at the scene of the accident, unless the condition is recognised and artificial respiration can be given immediately. For example, a patient was injured during a rugby game and sustained a fracture dislocation of C_2. A doctor at the ground had a beaver respirator in his car and was able to give artificial respiration until the patient reached hospital. The patient survived, the lesion became slightly incomplete and the patient was able to breathe unaided and was rehabilitated to life in a wheelchair.

Where the injury occurs at C_4 the patient usually manages to reach hospital on a partially funcioning diaphragm. Most lesions then ascend a segment when a ventilator becomes necessary. The lesion descends in the majority of cases and the patient finally manages to breathe unaided.

TREATMENT OF THE PATIENT WITH A LESION AT C_4

The patient with a complete lesion at C_4 has no motor power in the arms, trunk or legs. The major muscles remaining innervated are the upper portion of the trapezius and sternomastoid supplied by the accessory nerve, and platysma supplied by the facial nerve. There is complete loss of sensation, bladder, bowel and sexual function, and vasomotor control. As a result of the paralysis of the vasoconstrictors there is a marked vasodilatation initially. This causes blockage of the nasal air passages which adds to the difficulties of respiration without a tracheostomy. This phenomenon, known as Guttmann's sign, is often present in patients with lower cervical lesions also.

When the stage of spinal shock is over spasticity and rigidity of muscle develops, the limbs becoming predominantly spastic in extension. Physical rehabilitation is limited to training the vasomotor system to enable the patient to lead a wheelchair life and to teach him control of the power-drive chair. Although various activities are open to him by using a mouthstick, he is not capable of any degree of independence. Special equipment is needed for those patients who return home, and the relatives require expert training.

Physiotherapy during the acute stage

Chest therapy is vital and has been described in Chapter 5. Treatment will be needed every 2 hours at least, if not every hour, for the first 24–48 hours. It is advisable to continue daily postural drainage for several months as a prophylactic measure once the acute stage is over. For patients with a tendency to chest infection this should be continued throughout life. If a patient with a lesion at this level develops a head cold, he should remain in bed for a day or two to prevent secretions dripping down into the chest when the patient is vertical.

To minimise the effect of the extensor spasticity the position of the arms is important. From the first day the correct position is adduction of the shoulder, 45° flexion or mid position of the elbow, extension of the wrist, and flexion of the fingers.

When the fracture is healed, training for the Vasomotor system must be taken very slowly. An abdominal binder is often a help for the first few weeks to minimise pooling of the blood in the splanchnic vessels.

PHYSICAL REHABILITATION

The power-drive chair

Most patients at this level will need a semireclining, standard or junior power-drive chair. The control of the chair will need to be either with the chin, by pushing a small sensitive lever in the appropriate direction, or by two electronically controlled 'puff and suck' tubes in the mouth. A transit chair will also be needed as the power-drive chair is heavy to dismantle and put in a car.

Position of the patient in the wheelchair

The patient has no muscles with which to save himself, therefore his position in the chair must be carefully checked for safety and stability and to ensure that there are no factors likely to irritate his spasticity.

A semireclining chair assists both stability and respiration, particularly if the diaphragm remains partially paralysed. The arms need to be adequately supported to reduce spasticity and to minimise the strain on the shoulder joints. A tray makes a useful support, or the forearms and hands can be supported on a cushion on the lap.

PHYSIOTHERAPY

Once the patient is up treatment is directed towards:

1. Maintaining balance in the chair.
2. Reducing spasticity.
3. Hypertrophy of the innervated muscles.
4. Control of the power-drive chair.

Balance in the chair

Balance exercises in the chair are carried out in front of the mirror to help the patient (a) become aware of his position in space and (b) use his head and shoulders to maintain his equilibrium, especially when moving over uneven ground.

1. The therapist sits the patient away from the back of the chair and if necessary reclines the backrest to a larger angle to give more room for the exercise. The therapist finds the balance point and the patient tries to hold the position by moving his head and using trapezius.

2. The patient sits back in the chair, leaning against the backrest and facing the mirror. By flexing the head quickly and then lifting it quickly, the patient can learn to 'bounce' his shoulders away from the backrest. Having bounced the upper trunk away from the chair, the patient side flexes his head, and his upper trunk moves a few inches to one side. Once learnt this manoeuvre is invaluable as it aids stability when the chair is being moved. This may require a great deal of practise but it is well worth the effort involved.

Reduction of spasticity

Spasticity may be reduced by reflex-inhibiting postures on the mat, by careful positioning in bed at night, by standing and possibly by periods in a heated pool.

Standing

The therapist can stand the patient with a high lesion in plaster splints as described for patients with lower cervical lesions. Alternatively, the tilt table is useful for these patients as they have insufficient motor power to assist in maintaining their own standing position.

The patient stands for only 2 or 3 minutes the first day. This is increased to two periods of the same duration the second day. Subsequently the time is increased a few minutes only per day until the patient can stand for about 20 minutes. It is helpful to do this daily whilst training the vasomotor response, but afterwards the patient stands two or three times a week. If possible a relative is taught the technique so that the patient can continue to stand at home.

Swimming

When the patient is well used to being up in the chair and if he is keen to try, the heated pool may help the spasticity and give an overall feeling of well-being. In spite of the almost total paralysis, movement through the water can be achieved on the back by moving the head from side to side.

Hypertrophy of the innervated muscles

Hypertrophy of the few remaining muscles can be achieved with quite astonishing results.

OCCUPATIONAL THERAPY

The patient with the ultra-high lesion can learn to use various mouth sticks to type, turn pages, paint and play certain games. A platform can be fitted at a convenient height so that the patient can pick out and replace the mouth sticks required. Several environmental control systems are available which enable the completely paralysed patient to operate a selection of appliances in his environment (Maling, 1963). This is done by means of a switch, activated by the lightest touch, for example, of the chin, head or breath. The patient can for example put out the light, open the front door and turn on and tune the television. These patients can use a specially adapted phone and may have the incentive and ability to use an electronically operated typewriter, such as that produced by Possum or a computer (see p. 84).

HANDLING THE PATIENT

To lift the patient in the chair

This lift to relieve pressure has already been described (see p. 59).

To turn the patient

1. Cross one ankle over the other in the direction of the turn.

2. Turn the shoulders by putting one arm, for example the right, across the chest to hang down on the left side and pull the left shoulder back.

3. The therapist thrusts her arms underneath the buttocks until she can grip the anterior superior iliac spine, if possible. *The arms are kept close together*: the heavier the patient the closer the arms need to be.

4. Turn the buttocks and at the same time pull them back into the middle of the bed. The 'bounce' of the mattress can be utilised to flip the patient over.

To transfer the patient from chair to bed or car

The easiest method is by the cervical lift through standing as shown on page 122. Lift the patient and lower into the car seat in the manoeuvres already described. Hold the patient round the shoulders with one hand ensuring that his trunk and head are flexed well forwards. Lift the legs in and swivel the patient round with the other hand.

To get out reverse this procedure.

Car seats should be leather or plastic so that the patient slides easily.

To sit the patient up in bed

Facing the patient, hook one arm through the patient's nearside arm and place the other arm behind his shoulders. Pull and lift into the sitting position. The patient can assist the movement by bringing the head forward at the same time as the therapist beings to lift.

The sitting position can be maintained with minimum effort if the head and shoulders are kept well forward so that the centre of gravity is in front of the hip joints. If the patient has extensor spasticity, outwardly rotate the legs and flex the knees.

HANDLING THE WHEELCHAIR

To push up a kerb

Tip the chair on to its rear wheels by pressing down on the chair handles and one of the tipping levers.

Push the chair on the rear wheels until the front wheels are over the kerb.

Lower the chair onto the front wheels and push the rear wheels up the kerb.

To push down a kerb

Tilt the chair on to its rear wheels and push down the curb on the rear wheels only. Or, if the patient is large and heavy or excessively nervous, turn the chair round and allow the rear wheels to descend first.

To put the chair in the boot of the car

Take out the cushion and remove the footplates if necessary. Check that the brakes are on. With the side of the chair facing the operator hold onto the cross bars or the wheels. Tip the chair up onto the thighs and pivot it into the boot.

The wheels are usually placed to the back of the boot. Deep boots entail lifting the chair the depth of the boot before it can be taken out. Therefore, unless two chairs need to be carried, a boot in which the floor is level with the door is more convenient.

PERMANENT CARE

It is a tribute to the medical social workers, to the social services and particularly to relatives that so many of the patients with high lesions return to their own homes. Some patients have large families where the strain of caring for the disabled person is spread between several members. In other cases there is only one relative available. Some depend on maximum social support, others accept only a little help.

Patients with additional problems may need permanent hospital care. Others may have no suitable relative young and fit enough to cope with the full-time care needed. Some of these patients may be able to pay for the necessary assistance, others will need to go into long-term care in homes with heavy nursing wards.

The person who is to care for the very high lesion at home needs special training and should spend a minimum of a week at the hospital before the patient is discharged. She will need to learn how to handle the patient and the wheelchair, how to dress the patient and attend to the bladder and bowels. It is also important for her to see what the patient can do for himself and how best she can help him achieve even minimum independence.

Equipment

Beds

An Egerton turning bed and/or a ripple mattress is usually required for home use, but this will depend upon the size and age of the patient and relative. These aids do not *negate* the necessity to turn but either lengthen the period between turns or facilitate the turn itself. The young relative may prefer to turn the patient manually. Beds are available which raise the patient from supine to the sitting position. Where a turning bed is not required such a bed may be of great value in the home. It relieves the relatives of the effort normally involved in raising and lowering the patient. In some cases and with suitable adaptions, the patient may be able to operate the bed himself, thus achieving a small measure of independence.

Hoists

Since a hoist is cumbersome to have in the house some young relatives prefer to lift through standing. Others could not manage without a hoist.

The Split Hammock sling is recommended. This sling is completely safe for patients with high cervical lesions and can be removed during the day so that the patient does not have to sit on it.

Hoists are available to get in and out of the car but are often cumbersome and bulky to use. A simple hoist which fits over the roof of the car is made by S. Birvill & Son, engineers and manufacturers of elastic invalid hoists, 143, Hesham Road, Walton-on-Thames, Surrey.

Mechanisms are available which enable the patient *in* the wheelchair to be lifted either into the area of the passengers' seat or into the rear of a hatchback car or van.

14

The incomplete spinal lesion

GENERAL INTRODUCTION

The term 'incomplete lesion' encompasses all patients with some sparing of neural activity below the level of the lesion.

There has been a considerable increase in the number of patients with incomplete spinal cord lesions over the past 10 years. On average, 50% of patients in a spinal unit will have some sparing which may be as little as a flicker in one muscle, or joint position sense or there may be substantial functional recovery. An improved awareness of the nature of spinal injury has led to more efficient management of the patient at the site of the accident and subsequently on admission to a general hospital.

Incomplete lesions can result from either traumatic or pathological causes. The latter category includes those patients with:

— vascular accidents
— carcinoma
— transverse myelitis.

SYNDROMES

No two lesions will be identical. The pathology will always be different because of the complex nature of the spinal cord. However certain types are referred to as syndromes. These include:

— central cord syndrome
— Brown-Séquard syndrome
— anterior cord syndrome.

Central cord syndrome

Cause

This type of lesion usually results from a hyper-extension injury to the cervical spine. It is more commonly found in the older age groups, and is thought to be associated with the presence of spondylitic changes. As there may be no evidence of a fracture, this lesion may be difficult to diagnose. Computerised tomography may provide extra information.

Clinical picture

Damage occurs to the central part of the cord, the long tracts remaining relatively intact.

The general clinical picture is of:

— disproportionately more motor involvement in the upper extremities than in the lower.
— bladder dysfunction, often with urinary retention.
— varying degrees of sensory impairment (Fig. 14.1).

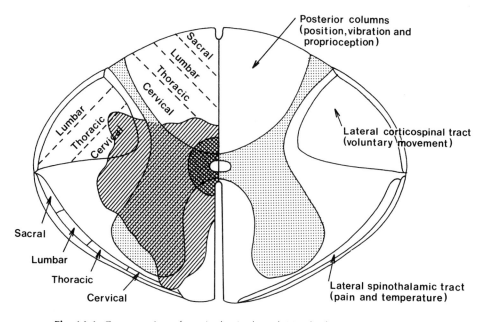

Fig. 14.1 Cross-section of cervical spinal cord. Hatched areas represent a zone of central haemorrhage ▨ and surrounding oedema ///// : the impingement on pathways, especially central cervical fibres, in part subserving upper extremity function, is readily apparent (after Morse, 1982).

Motor deficit

At the level of the lesion there will be damage to the anterior horn cells resulting in a flaccid paralysis of those muscles supplied from this level. The gradual wasting of these muscles gives rise to the fairly typical picture of the central cord lesion. The development of contractures and/or painful joints of the upper limbs will remain a very real danger throughout all stages of rehabilitation.

The hands may be relatively uninvolved but without the background of proximal stability, maximal function cannot be achieved.

In other cases, the hands may be paralysed, when swelling may occur due to the effect of gravity. This can lead to the development of stiff and painful joints.

Depending on the severity of the lesion, the patient will demonstrate some degree of motor deficit in the trunk and lower limbs which is characterised by the presence of spasticity.

The majority of these patients will achieve an independent gait with or without the use of walking aids.

Sensory deficit

This is extremely variable ranging from severe sensory loss to virtually no impairment.

The disability of these patients is often under-estimated. The patient's ability to walk makes him appear less disabled, whereas without the use of his arms, he may be more handicapped than the chairbound paraplegic.

Brown-Séquard syndrome

Cause

Damage occurs to one side of the cord from a closed injury, a stab wound or other penetrating trauma.

Clinical picture

Motor deficit

Motor loss occurs on the same side as the lesion due to destruction of the pyramidal tracts.

The lower motor lesion, resulting from damage to the anterior horn cells at the level of the lesion, will be particularly significant at the lumbar or sacral enlargements.

Sensory deficit

Destruction of the posterior column results in loss of position sense, vibration and tactile discrimination below the level of the lesion on the affected side.

Destruction of the lateral spinothalamic tract causes loss of sensation of pain and temperature *on the side opposite to the lesion*. As the fibres entering this tract do not cross for several segments, the upper level of this sensory loss is likely to be a few segments below the level of the lesion. Fibres entering the cord at the level of the lesion may be involved before they cross causing a narrow zone of similar pain and temperature loss *on the same side*.

(Most patients with incomplete lesions will present with some asymmetry whilst not fulfilling the exact criteria of the Brown-Séquard syndrome described above.)

Anterior spinal cord syndrome

Cause

Traumatic. This syndrome often results from a forced flexion, compression injury which can occur in diving accidents.

Non-traumatic. The anterior cord syndrome may result from anterior spinal artery thrombosis, spinal cord angioma or aortic aneuryectomy.

Clinical picture

Motor deficit

Depending on the severity there will be motor impairment below the level of the lesion which will range from total loss of motor control to more minor degrees of dysfunction.

Sensory loss

There will be disturbance of pain and temperature sensation but proprioception will remain relatively intact.

Secondary carcinoma

Clinical picture

This will depend on the site and size of the mass affecting the spinal cord.

Transverse myelitis

Definition. Inflammation of the spinal cord, usually involving both the grey and the white matter, in a considerable part of its transverse extent. When the lesion is limited longitudinally to a few segments, it is described as transverse myelitis (Brain).

The cause of the inflammation may remain undiagnosed in many cases.

Clinical picture

This will depend on the level at which the inflammation occurs.

TREATMENT

General comments

It is essential for all persons involved in the rehabilitation of the patient with an incomplete spinal cord injury to assess the disability of each patient as it relates to that individual and not to compare him with other patients, especially those with complete lesions.

As with any patient, factors such as age, physical proportions, motivation and previous occupation must be taken into account in the rehabilitation programme.

Considerable progress has been made in the understanding and treatment of spasticity which will benefit patients with incomplete lesions.

Psychological factors

Obviously, with both complete and incomplete lesions, the psychological factors resulting from such a devastating injury, have to be taken into account throughout all stages of rehabilitation.

With the incomplete lesion, there may be a problem in the patient coming to terms with his disability. Being incomplete, prognosis is ill-defined, and it is particularly difficult, even for those with a substantial functional recovery, to accept less than 100% normality.

If surrounded by patients with complete lesions, it is easy to consider the patient with an incomplete lesion fortunate because he has some sparing. Although this is true, even those patients making a good recovery may still be unable to return to their normal life-style.

The physiotherapist, because of her close contact with the patient, may be the one chosen as 'confidante' by both the patient and his relatives. It is important that she allows them to express their fears and/or frustrations while offering constructive advice. Where more professional counselling is thought to be required, the patient and/or relatives should be encouraged to talk to their social worker or in some cases a clinical psychologist.

Basic principles of treatment

Basic principles include:

— rehabilitation of the body as a whole to train balance, co-ordination and control.
— inhibition and/or facilitation of all affected muscle groups to allow them to function on a background of more normal postural tone.
— the stronger muscle groups should not be allowed to dominate movement as this will further inhibit the affected groups and may well exacerbate spasticity.

The Bobath concept embraces these basic principles. By observation, assessment and handling the patient in such a way as to bring about a normalisation of postural tone, the patient's problems are identified and treatment planned to meet the specific needs of the individual patient.

There can be no set routine in terms of an exercise programme, mat work or gait re-education. Each treatment is viewed as a re-assessment of the patient's status and treatment adapted accordingly.

Normal movement

The treatment described in this chapter is based upon an accurate and extensive knowledge of normal movement, an understanding of which is essential for the successful treatment of any patient with neurological damage.

Normal movement depends upon a central nervous system that is able to receive, integrate and respond to the sensory information it receives from both exteroceptors, e.g. visual or tactile, and interoceptors, e.g. muscle spindles or golgi tendon organs.

The mechanism which produces this integrated response is referred to as the normal postural reflex mechanism (Bobath).

The essential requirements for a normal postural reflex mechanism are:

1. A normal sensory-motor feedback system
2. Normal postural tone
3. Reciprocal innervation
4. Righting and equilibrium reactions.

1. Normal sensory-motor feedback system

Where the central nervous system is intact, movement occurs in response to stimuli. This is dependent not only on normal sensation, but also on normal selective movement patterns which allow an appropriate response. Patients with incomplete spinal cord injuries will have varying degrees of sensory loss.

If sensory stimuli from muscles, tendons and joint receptors are disturbed, this will affect the initiation, guidance and control of movement.

Where spasticity is present, the patient will receive abnormal sensations from his spastic muscles and immobile joints. He will feel resistance to movement and this sensory state, when interpreted by the brain, will result in increased effort to overcome this resistance. The extra effort further increases the spasticity and the patient's feeling of resistance to movement.

Abnormal sensation will inevitably limit successful rehabilitation as the sensory-motor feedback system is impaired.

2. Normal postural tone

Normal postural tone develops in response to gravity. It must be high enough to withstand gravity and yet low enough to allow mobility. It must be adaptable to respond to the body's requirements, maintaining stability and allowing function, e.g. writing requires distal mobility at the wrist and fingers and proximal stability of the trunk and shoulders.

Adaptations of postural tone are automatic and occur in response to functional objectives.

3. Reciprocal innervation

This is the interplay between opposing muscle groups permitting both dynamic co-contraction for postural stability and controlled graded movements for function. For example when taking food to the mouth, the flexors and extensors of the elbow work together reciprocally, on a background of dynamic co-contraction at the shoulder girdle to allow a smooth functional movement to be performed successfully.

Any disturbance in the balance of postural tone for example by spasticity or motor loss will interfere with reciprocal innervation.

4. Righting and equilibrium reactions

Righting reactions. Automatic reactions occur in response to alteration of body alignment. These are precipitated by the head, trunk or limbs to enable the body to regain the midline. The righting reactions form a basis for all gross activities and are an integral part of all sequences of movement.

Equilibrium reactions. These are automatic postural adjustments which occur in response to displacement of the body's centre of gravity. Equilibrium reactions vary from minute adjustments which occur throughout daily life, to the gross saving reactions which come into play when all else has failed.

When standing still, the muscles of the feet are constantly making minute adjustments to maintain the body's centre of gravity over its base. This activity is accentuated if the base is narrowed, and even more so when standing on one leg.

Equilibrium reactions may be demonstrated by either moving the base or displacing the body away from its centre of gravity. The greater the insecurity, the more pronounced the reaction, e.g. when gently displacing the centre of gravity backwards the activity in the dorsi-flexors of the feet becomes more pronounced, and as the force applied is increased, the arms are outstretched. As the body becomes unable to cope with the displacing force stepping backwards occurs to restore the centre of gravity over its base. If a sudden force is applied of such magnitude that the body is unable to adjust and falls, protective extension of the arms occurs in whatever direction is required to protect the head and face from injury.

Equilibrium reactions occur throughout the whole body but they are effective only on a background of normal postural tone.

An awareness of the normal postural reflex mechanism is essential in the understanding of normal movement and its subsequent application to the treatment of the patient with incomplete spinal cord injury.

TREATMENT OF THE ACUTE LESION IN BED

During the acute phase physiotherapy includes active and passive movements to all affected limbs. Correct positioning is essential for the reasons stated in Chapter 3 and in particular to minimise the dominance of stereotyped spasticity. Muscle charts are necessary to monitor recovery and are revised at regular intervals.

Positioning

The position of the patient with an incomplete lesion will be the same as that for the complete lesion, except where severe spasticity is a complicating factor. If the extensor aspect of the patient's body is in contact with the bed, as is the case even when on his 'side' on the Egerton-Stoke Mandeville Electric Turning Bed, a stimulus is provided for him to push against which exacerbates the extensor spasticity. In order to control the spasticity in these cases, it may be necessary to use a pillow and sandbags to support the fracture and keep the patient in side-lying instead of using the turning bed.

The 'frog position', where the hips are abducted, laterally rotated and flexed to approximately 40°, can be used to break up severe extensor spasticity. Patients positioned in this way to control the extensor tone should be closely monitored for any increase in flexor tone, as it is possible to reverse completely the pattern of spasticity.

Movements

The importance of movement for these patients is well recognised, but it is the way in which the movements are performed which is of special concern. In all cases, the movements are considered active in the sense that the patient is attempting to accomplish the required movement with the assistance of the physiotherapist. The patient must be totally involved in understanding the movement required of him and give his total co-operation and attention to this end.

The maintenance of joint range must not become a routine procedure which can be done without thought. If the physiotherapist has a good understanding of normal movement, she will appreciate changes in tone and, by her handling, modify this tone before taking the limb through normal joint range. If movements are performed in this way, with close communication between patient and therapist, there will be less danger of trauma and of the joints becoming painful and contracted.

Time spent mobilising the patient should be a learning experience for him, enabling him to use his recovering muscles in a normal pattern of movement thereby preventing early and perhaps unnecessary compensation.

Effort during movement should be avoided where spasticity is present. The physiotherapist gives sufficient guidance and assistance to the patient to reduce to a minimum the effort required to perform the movement. This is particularly important where spasticity may jeopardize stability at the fracture site. Some patients may be particularly sensitive to any stimulus, even removal of the bed clothes prior to doing the movements, and with cervical lesions, it may be necessary for another therapist to support the shoulders to eliminate excessive movement around the fracture site.

In the majority of patients extensor spasticity is the dominant pattern. This may involve the arms as well as the trunk and legs of a patient with a high cervical lesion. A combination of both flexor and extensor spasticity frequently occurs and movement initially may be from one total pattern to the other.

In those cases where there is severe extensor spasticity, it may be necessary initially to move the limbs into the total flexor pattern, in order to have any effect on the predominant extension. After breaking up the total extensor synergy it is important to work recovering muscles out of any stereotyped pattern. For example with the leg flexed, the patient is encouraged to use any active hip flexion with adduction and medial rotation, and when moving into extension this should incorporate abduction and lateral rotation — always maintaining control to avoid an extensor thrust.

EARLY MOBILISATION

As with the complete lesion, the length of time spent in bed will depend on whether there has been surgical intervention.

Depending on the degree of cord damage, it may be necessary to retrain:

— vasomotor control
— pressure consciousness
— postural sensibility.

As there is significant asymmetry in most cases which results in postural scoliosis, the retraining of postural sensibility is vital.

Factors influencing the choice of chair and accessories

The chapter on wheelchairs, including the positioning of the patient in the chair, also applies to the patients with incomplete spinal cord lesions. In addition, there are certain other factors which will influence the choice of chair for these patients.

1. Asymmetrical trunk control

Adjustable arm rests may be used to correct the position of patients with postural scoliosis. The majority of patients will lean to their less affected side. If the arm rest on this side is elevated, symmetry will be restored and the risk of permanent deformity reduced.

2. Recovering motor power in the legs

Patients who retain or regain relatively good use of the legs, for example those with a central cord lesion, can use their legs to manoeuvre the chair. The wheelchair which is 3 inches lower than the standard model allows the feet to reach the ground, and makes pushing the chair easier.

It is important that the patient sits with the buttocks well back in the seat, flexing at the hips to propel the chair. A padded board or a wheelchair cushion may be positioned against the backrest to prevent the patient leaning backwards in the chair. If this is allowed to occur, the patient will inevitably propel the chair backwards using and thereby exacerbating his extensor spasticity (Fig. 14.2a & b).

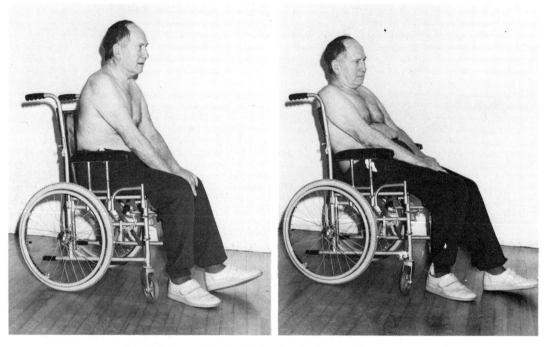

Fig. 14.2 Propelling the chair using the legs. (a) Correct position. (b) Incorrect position.

Mobilisation of the trunk

Spasticity may be exacerbated in all patients with incomplete lesions by compensation of the head and trunk for the more apparent distal problems. In order to prevent this, it is important to work proximally for modification of tone distally.

The value of active or passive trunk rotation is well recognised as a means of inhibiting spasticity.

The majority of patients with central cord lesions will have a marked degree of immobility of the head and trunk due to the lack of movement and subsequent balance reactions of the arms.

Movement of the trunk against the limbs

Proximal movement against an inhibited distal point is a useful way of reducing spasticity. For example, starting with the patient sitting with his arms around the physiotherapist or supported on a platform of suitable height, the trunk is moved from side to side and/or forwards and backwards ensuring that the weight is forwards over the feet during the movement (Fig. 14.3a & b). As a result of the proximal movement of the trunk against the inhibited position of the arms, spasticity will be reduced in both arms and legs.

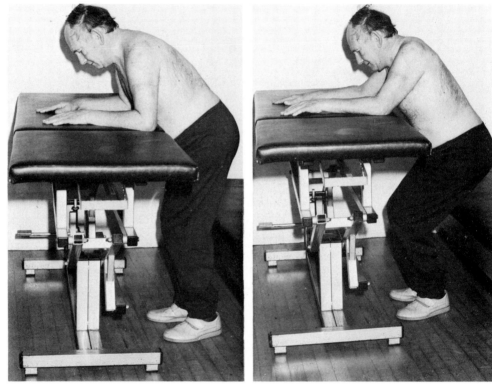

a   b

Fig. 14.3 (a & b) Movement of trunk against limbs.

Improving joint range at the shoulders

Treatment for improving the joint range of the shoulders is more effective when the patient is controlling his own movement by moving the trunk against the inhibited limbs. With the arm correctly supported at the shoulder and the patient moving from lying to sitting and back to lying, elongation of the trunk side flexors with rotation will occur which will further inhibit increased tone in the upper limb.

For this to be effective, the shoulder must be fully supported in the axilla and the arm held in lateral rotation.

Pelvic tilt

In many patients with incomplete lesions there is impairment of pelvic tilt.

Those patients with flexor spasticity of the lower limbs will have an increased lumbar lordosis with anterior pelvic tilt to compensate for the flexion at the hips. In the majority of patients with cervical lesions, the lumbar spine becomes flattened with posterior pelvic tilt due to the more frequently found extensor spasticity of the legs.

Treatment of this problem should not be confined to pelvic tilt exercises in supine. Correction should be given in all relevant positions, e.g. sitting, kneeling and standing, and the patient made aware of his improved posture and how to correct it himself.

Gymnastic ball

Treatment using the gymnastic ball was originally devised by Klein-Vogelbach and has been adapted for use in neurological conditions.

The ball which is made of resilient hard plastic comes in various sizes and may be used with good effect in the treatment of some patients with incomplete spinal cord injuries.

The choice of size depends upon the reason for which the ball is being used and the physical proportions of the patient.

The ball is useful:

— as a means of inhibition and proximal mobilisation where there is excessive spasticity
— in retraining balance reactions and co-ordination thereby improving body awareness
— in giving controlled strengthening exercises where weakness of specific muscle groups is apparent.

It is essential that the patient is totally confident and unafraid. If the patient is frightened, not only will the treatment be ineffective, but it may cause a significant increase in spasticity and therefore prove to be detrimental.

EARLY WEIGHT-BEARING

Early weight-bearing is encouraged with the physiotherapist controlling the hips and knees as necessary. Where there is severe motor deficit, plaster back slabs may be of value initially to enable the patient to gain better trunk control. As the patient becomes more proficient, only one slab need be used, perhaps alternately on each leg to allow the patient to use his recovering muscles actively.

Where there is motor sparing, the patient uses his motor power in all functional activities, e.g. the chosen method to transfer would always be with the feet down.

Early weight-bearing of the upper limbs is also included for patients with cervical lesions, particularly those with central cord lesions. Where there is poor motor control, great care is taken to ensure that the shoulder joint in particular is well protected and adequately supported. It is essential to ensure weight-bearing in a normal movement pattern with trunk elongation and lateral rotation of the arms and not allow medial rotation and adduction at the shoulder. If the patient complains of pain or has limited range of movement at the wrist, weight-bearing may be used as a means of gentle mobilisation within the painfree range.

NORMAL MOVEMENT IN RELATION TO FUNCTION

Muscles do not work in isolation. Where there is muscle imbalance, it is most important to strengthen the individual muscles as a part of normal movement.

Throughout all stages of rehabilitation, treatment is aimed at improving the patient's functional abilities without the use of unnecessary compensation.

The teaching of activities of daily living should involve the maximum use of the more affected muscle groups, the physiotherapist giving as much assistance as is necessary for the patient to experience a normal sequence of movement. This will only be possible on a background of normal postural tone. The handling skills of the physiotherapist in facilitating and/or inhibiting tone are of paramount importance.

GAIT ANALYSIS AND RE-EDUCATION

The patient's problems are identified by observation and handling, and a course of treatment planned for the re-education of gait.

Gait may be broadly divided into four phases:

— transfer of weight onto one leg
— simultaneous release of opposite leg
— step through phase
— transfer of weight onto forward leg.

The patient may have impairment of all four phases or have more specific problems with any one phase.

The different problems which occur are too numerous and diverse to permit a standardised approach to treatment. However there are certain preparatory steps which are essential for the patient to learn prior to commencing gait re-education.

1. Standing balance with the body in correct alignment and with the weight taken throughout the whole surface of the feet.
2. Standing without using the arms. If this is impossible, the patient is encouraged to use his arms for balance only. If the patient learns to push down with the hands in front, the weight is brought forwards over the ball of the foot thereby eliciting an extensor thrust.
3. Hip and knee control. It is essential that the patient has adequate control at the hip to prevent hyper-extension of the knee.
4. Stability of the trunk and pelvis with weight transference to either side and release of the non-weight-bearing leg.
5. Weight transference to either leg in step standing.
6. Stepping through without excessive use of the trunk.

A means of enabling the patient to walk when he may otherwise have insufficient hip and/or knee control is by the physiotherapist using a stool on wheels. The physiotherapist sits on the stool, in front of the patient with the patient's hands on her shoulders (Fig. 14.4). This enables the therapist to have sufficient control at each phase of gait to facilitate a more normal gait pattern.

Obviously, the ability of the patient to attain a normal gait pattern will depend on his neurological deficit. For example, if a patient requires a long leg caliper on one leg, he will be unable to step through without hitching at the hip.

Orthoses

The choice of orthosis will depend upon the degree of paralysis and the severity of spasticity. Not only the rehabilitation staff, but also the patient must be involved in this choice. Unless the patient believes that the orthosis will benefit him, and is prepared to use it, there is no value in supplying one.

There has been considerable improvement in the orthoses available with particular emphasis on their cosmetic appearance. The

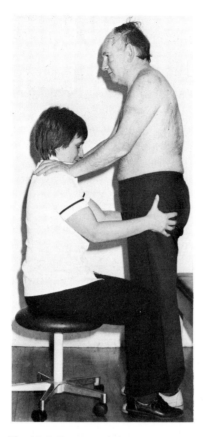

Fig. 14.4 Position of physiotherapist using stool on wheels.

lightweight, moulded orthoses are often appropriate for patients with flaccid paralysis and may also be used for some patients with spasticity.

To assess the benefit of a below knee orthosis, a bandage can be used to maintain the foot in dorsiflexion. Where spasticity is present, the bandage must hold the foot in eversion as well as dorsiflexion to inhibit the spastic invertors (Fig. 14.5, a, b, c). Not only does this allow the physiotherapist to assess the patient's gait with the appropriate correction, but it also indicates if the patient is likely to develop proximal spasticity in response to the corrective device on his foot.

Patients with incomplete spinal cord injury show varied problems necessitating different orthoses which can range from full leg calipers to a single below-knee splint. Great care is taken with selection and the patient must be assessed at regular intervals following discharge from hospital to ensure that the orthosis remains appropriate to his needs.

Walking aids

Where possible the aid should be used to assist balance rather than as a means of support.

Crutches, a rollator or the paient's own wheelchair is preferred to a frame, as with these aids, the patient is able to obtain a greater degree of hip and trunk extension and in consequence a more normal walking pattern. With the frame in the forward position, prior to the patient taking a step, flexion and retraction occur at the hips thereby increasing the danger of hyper-extension of the knees.

If either one or two sticks are required, they should be slightly higher than is usually prescribed. This prevents the patient using them for excessive support and initiating walking by means of trunk flexion and trunk side-flexion.

TREATMENT OF THE PATIENT WITH CARCINOMA

The prognosis of these patients must be borne in mind when planning their treatment. When the prognosis is good, the patient should be treated along the lines already indicated.

If the prognosis is poor, it is essential that the relatives be involved from the beginning as it may be desirable to allow the patient to return home as soon as possible to give him the maximum time in his familiar environment.

The patient and relatives are taught the easiest methods for

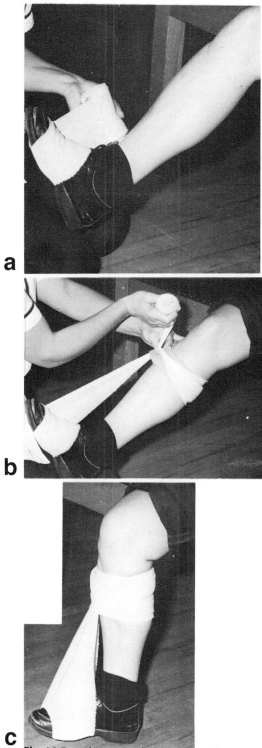

Fig. 14.5   (a, b & c) Application of bandage to maintain foot in dorsiflexion and eversion.

performing the activities of daily living which allow adequate support for the patient and produce the least strain on the relatives.

Wherever possible, a home visit is carried out in conjunction with the occupational therapist and a representative of the social services to ensure every assistance is given to the family.

15

Spinal cord injury in children

The incidence of spinal cord injury in children under 13 years is much smaller than in teenagers and adults. Children sustain their injuries through road traffic accidents, whether in a vehicle or as a pedestrian, diving and swimming accidents, gunshot wounds, and falls from heights.

Frequently there is no evidence of vertebral fracture or dislocation, although there may be severe spinal cord damage. It has been suggested (Burke, 1971) that through its elasticity and cartilaginous properties the spine of a young child can withstand gross distortion, especially in flexion and rotation, without fracturing bones. The spinal cord cannot stand the same degree of stretch, consequently traction results in cord damage.

The treatment of the initial injury and the overall plan of care and rehabilitation are the same for the child as for the adult. The necessary changes in rehabilitation result from the problems attendant upon continuing growth or the age and size of the child. The deviations from the treatment for adults are given below.

PHYSICAL REHABILITATION

There are no variations from the adult programme in the physiotherapy given to the child in bed. The changes that occur are in the later stages of rehabilitation.

THE WHEELCHAIR

It is important to see that the wheelchair is suitable, that it is not too big or too heavy, and that the child will be able to manipulate it skilfully.

POSTURAL SENSIBILITY

Children aged 3 years and over are given short periods of training sitting on the plinth in front of the mirror in the usual way. This is augmented for small children by play therapy on the mat. Games and activities involving the use of first one and then both hands are encouraged whilst the unassisted sitting position is maintained. Children under 3 years are usually treated daily on the mat only, but where possible a mirror is used to give the child the necessary visual feedback.

MAT WORK

The ability of the young child to sit up from lying down is very important as it releases the mother from going to the child early in the morning to sit him up in his cot to play. Where this activity has not been taught, the mother may continue to lift the child even when he is 5, 6 or 7 years of age.

To sit up from lying down on the mat:

1. Turn the upper trunk and left arm to the right (Fig. 15.1a).
2. Push up onto both elbows (Fig. 15.1b).
3. 'Walk' on the hands to the sitting position (Fig. 15.1c and d).

The child also is taught to turn over, to roll into the prone position and to move himself and his legs around on the mat.

MUSCLE STRENGTH

In order to prevent spinal deformity which occurs more readily in children than in adults, it is particularly important to hypertrophy the back muscles and latissimus dorsi.

DRESSING AND SELF-CARE

The child with spinal cord injury is taught to dress and wash at the same age as the able-bodied child. He is also taught as early as possible to look at his own legs for pressure marks, to put pillows between the legs when turning in bed, and to lift and move with care.

TRANSFERS

Chair to bed

It is easier and safer for the young child to get onto the bed forwards (see Ch. 11).

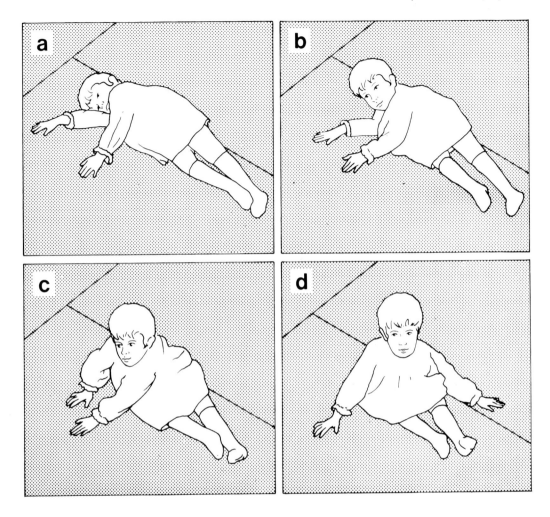

Fig. 15.1 Sitting up. Child with a complete lesion below T_{10}.

Chair to car

A sliding board may be necessary if the gap is too wide for the small child.

Chair to bath and chair to floor

The lifts involved are usually too great for a child. Stools of varying height can be used as steps for the child to get from his chair to the floor and back. A bath seat may be used in a similar way.

Chair to toilet

When transferring, the child will need to keep his feet on the footplates or have them propped on a solid stool of suitable height until his legs are long enough for his feet to reach the floor.

GAIT

Children usually take longer to learn the techniques involved, but generally prove much more efficient than adults, often being able to dispense with the wheelchair altogether. Where possible all three gaits are taught. The young child commences gait training as early as possible, i.e. 18 months.

Bone growth

If the child spends sufficient time on his feet, that is, at least 4 or more hours per day, growth defect will be kept to a minimum.

When balance in standing is good, children of preschool age can stand in the play group and at home to paint and play. This has the added psychological advantage of making the child, at least for a time, the same height as his fellows.

Long periods of weight-bearing also help to minimise the effect of osteoporosis and therefore of spontaneous fractures. The child with a brace and calipers must learn to lock and unlock the hip joints when standing if he is to be totally independent.

Equipment

At the commencement of gait training, plaster of Paris splints are made for the children in the same way as for adults.

Calipers

The calipers are obtained as quickly as possible. Knee joints are included in the calipers as soon as it is practical, that is, as soon as the child's leg is long enough to allow joints to be incorporated. It is important for the child to be able to stand and walk as required, and unless the child is very small, the weight of the straight caliper can cause pressure at the top of the leg when sitting down. Extensions are put in above and below the knee joints to allow for growth.

Brace

Most children with thoracic lesions above T_{12} will need a brace to prevent or correct spinal deformity. In most cases the brace will be attached to the calipers. If the brace is to be worn without the calipers the extensions with the hip joints must be part of the calipers not of the brace.

The therapist must check the equipment constantly and arrange for the frequent adjustments necessary to allow for the child's growth.

Chair to standing

His height prevents the young child from getting out of the chair onto his crutches using the forwards technique. The child can usually lift himself onto his feet by lifting on both armrests, or using the sideways method.

CHAIR MANOEUVRES

These should be learnt as for the adult, including rear wheel balance for the child of approximately 7 years and over. It is safer to teach a child to accomplish rear wheel balance safely than to have him try to do it without being taught.

CARE OF THE CHILD AT HOME

The mother or other relative who is in charge of the child at home will need to spend a week at the hospital with the child before discharge. It is essential that the mother learns in detail the care of the bladder, bowels and skin and to see how he walks and how to give him any necessary assistance. It is important also for the mother to see what the child can accomplish by himself, for example dressing, transfers, and to be taught how important it is that the child should continue his independence when home, even if he is slow at first.

Where possible, frequent visits home are encouraged during rehabilitation. After discharge from hospital, more frequent checkups are necessary for the growing child.

Education

The education of the physically handicapped child is of paramount importance. He must be enabled to make the best use of his brain since so many manual occupations will be impossible for him. The Education Act 1981 has introduced the principles of the integration of children with special educational needs with able-bodied children and the development of facilities to meet the special needs of handicapped children. It is desirable that, after spinal cord injury, children should return to normal schools and play groups when their initial period of rehabilitation is concluded. They will then integrate at an early age with able-bodied children and will also have the same chance to achieve the necessary qualifications for higher education. It is encouraging that more schools are welcoming the child back to school after becoming handicapped and are making the necessary alterations to school buildings.

SECONDARY VERTEBRAL DEFORMITIES

Various intrinsic factors contribute to the development of spinal deformities in children and adolescents:

1. The level of the lesion—the child is at great risk where the abdominal and back muscles are paralysed.

2. Disturbance of the muscle balance of the trunk—this may occur through spasticity.

3. The younger the patient the more prone he is to deformity because of continuing growth.

4. Para-articular ossification of the hip joint causing limitation in flexion may result in a scoliosis if one hip takes maximum pressure, or in a lumbar kyphosis if both hips are affected.

Spinal deformity seriously affects sitting balance and therefore independence. There are also the dangers of pressure sores due to unequal weight distribution and impairment of respiratory function if the scoliosis is severe.

In order to prevent secondary deformities some advocate that, until they are fully grown, children should sit for very short periods only. The majority of the time should be spent standing in brace and calipers or lying down. Trolleys with large wheels enable children to lie prone and propel themselves. Small self-propelling standing frames can be used as an alternative to crutch walking in order to maintain weight-bearing in the erect position for longer periods.

Prevention of spinal deformity

1. The treatment, correct positioning and quality of physiotherapy in the early weeks after injury influence the development of all deformities.

2. The back muscles must be hypertrophied as far as possible to prevent deformity through muscle weakness.

3. The patient must be adequately braced if there is the slightest suspicion of lateral or anteroposterior deformity.

4. The posture must be constantly corrected and observation maintained for the earliest sign of pelvic tilt in the sitting position.

5. A careful watch must be kept on the spine at all stages of treatment, and after discharge at checkups.

16

Complications

CONTRACTURES

Contractures introduce delays and complications into the patient's programme of rehabilitation. It is the direct responsibility of the therapist and nursing staff to prevent their occurrence.

Causes of contractures

1. Incorrect positioning in bed or incorrect posture in the wheel-chair.
2. Inadequate physiotherapy.
3. Spasticity.

It is difficult to separate these three closely linked factors in relation to the formation of a contracture.

Conservative treatment of established contractures

1. Passive movements, including accessory joint play.
2. Prolonged passive stretching.
3. Active exercises.
4. Splinting.
5. Passive and active exercises in a heated pool.
6. Ice therapy and ultrasound.

Passive movements

Passive movements are always given at every treatment in addition to any other methods employed. In conjunction with the passive movements a passive stretch is also given in the position of maximum correction.

Prolonged passive stretching

A prolonged passive stretch can be given for flexion contractures of the hips and knees and adduction contractures of the hips by strapping the limbs in the corrected position. *In bed* the corrective position is maintained by using pillows and padded straps. For example, when the knee flexors are contracted the legs are kept in extension with a strap over the knees. To avoid pressure, pillows are placed (a) under the lower legs to keep the heels off the bed, (b) between the knees to prevent the apposition of skin surfaces, and (c) over the knees, underneath the strap.

On the plinth

Adduction contractures. The patient lies supine on the plinth with pillows under his buttocks and trunk.

The legs are placed over the sides of the plinth with a pillow between the medial side of each knee and the plinth to prevent pressure.

Each knee is tied down and care is taken to see that the hip lies in lateral rotation (Fig. 16.1a).

Flexion contracture of the hips. The patient lies prone on the plinth. Two or three pillows are placed under the knees and similarly under the trunk, with a gap at the level of the hip joints. To avoid pressure a pillow is placed between the knees, and the toes must be over the end of the plinth (Fig. 16.1b). Correction is obtained by strapping the hips down to the plinth. The strap placed over a pillow on the sacrum is tightened gradually. Care must be taken to arrange the two groups of pillows so that the stretch is given to the hip flexors. If the space between the pillows is too wide the stretch merely increases the lumbar lordosis. The ankles can also be tied down with a padded strap if there are flexion contractures of the knees.

The stretch is normally maintained for 20–30 minutes.

Active exercises

Where the muscle groups are innervated hold-relax techniques are used to obtain relaxation of the contracted muscle groups, and resisted work is always given to the antagonists.

Splinting

To avoid excessive pressure it is advisable to make serial splints and

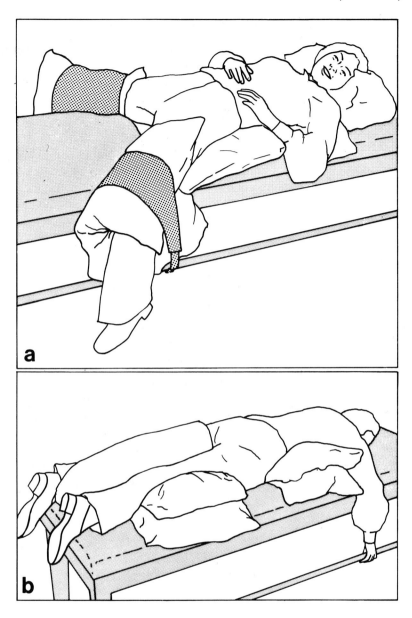

Fig. 16.1 Passive stretch. (a) For the adductor muscles. (b) For the hip flexor muscles.

not try to obtain maximum correction initially. The contracture may involve more than one joint. In this case, maximum correction is obtained firstly in the joint principally controlled by the major muscle involved. For example, where the elbow, wrist and fingers are flexed, biceps is the major muscle and maximum correction is given at the elbow joint.

Passive and active exercises in a heated pool

The hot water aids relaxation, and is especially beneficial if there is severe spasticity.

Ice therapy and ultrasound

Ice therapy and ultrasound are used as and where suitable.

'Constant attack' is the motto for dealing with contractures. Treatment needs to be carried out several times a day using a variety of methods. For example, contracted biceps tendons have been successfully treated by giving daily passive movements, active exercises, ice therapy, ultrasound and splinting; hip and knee flexion contractures by giving passive movements, passive stretching on the plinth, ice therapy and exercises in a heated pool.

Surgical treatment

When *no* improvement has occurred for approximately 6 weeks in spite of intensive therapy, the patient may be referred for surgery.

Release of the ileopsoas by ileopsoas myotomy (Michaelis, 1964), elongation of the Achilles tendon and obturator neurectomy to release the adductor muscles are useful surgical procedures in cases of severe contractures which have not responded to conservative methods. If the patient has strong spasticity as well as contractures other surgical procedures may be recommended (see pp. 226–227).

SPINAL DEFORMITIES

Development of spinal deformity

Any patient re-confined to bed for some time is in danger of developing contractures and may also develop a scoliosis. Children and adolescents are in particular danger because of continuing growth and extreme joint mobility.

When a patient spends a high proportion of time in an abnormal, incorrect posture for functional activities, convenience or comfort, deformities develop. Gross scoliosis or pelvic distortion will severely hamper the patient's rehabilitation and may prevent him from attaining complete independence or from functional weight-bearing.

Every effort must be made to prevent such deformities by correct positioning, muscle development and re-education of posture.

Distortion of the spine and pelvis through habitual abnormal postures

Examples

The following are some examples of abnormal postures commonly assumed by patients with spinal cord injury which can give rise to scoliosis and pelvic distortion.

In bed

A patient with a thoracic or lumbar lesion who is in bed for some time to heal a pressure sore, for example on the right trochanter, may be nursed on his back and left side only. All functional activities —washing, feeding and writing — may be done with the right hand and the patient will prop himself on his left elbow. This will involve habitual work for the right trunk side flexors. As a result the patient may develop a long C curve to the left.

Even if such a patient is being turned on his back and both sides, he may 'half sit up', propped on his elbow when on one side to use his dominant hand for functional activities. Again he may develop a long C curve to the opposite side.

The very active patient wanting to use his hands when spending long periods prone may develop an increased, or even gross lordosis. To prevent this, the pillows and packs under his head must be lowered, or removed for periods to allow him to work with his hands at a lower level.

In the wheelchair

A child constantly working at his desk in lateral flexion and possibly rotation may develop a scoliosis.

A child watching television or assuming a 'listening' posture, with his head always resting on the same hand and the elbow propped on the armrest, can produce a deformity in a similar way.

A patient constantly sitting with the same leg crossed over the other is at risk, as the maximum weight is always on one side, that is, on one ischium.

Where an ischiectomy has been performed on one side maximum weight will be taken on the opposite side and pelvic distortion may result. To redistribute the weight a hole can be cut in the cushion on the non-operated side if necessary.

Ischiectomies are often performed on both sides, even though only one side is affected, to prevent spinal deformity developing.

In standing

Increased lordosis occurs particularly in children and adolescents with lesions at T_{7-8} and above. This appears to be due to the extreme mobility of the joints and the lack of abdominal muscles.

Flattening of the lumbar curve occurs with patients with low thoracic lesions $T_{11}-L_1$ due to the imbalance between the innervated abdominal muscles and the paralysed sacrospinalis, illeopsoas and the muscles of the legs.

Increased forward tilt of the pelvis with lordosis develops in patients with lesions below L_3 through the overaction of ileopsoas and rectus femoris and the loss of innervation of the gluteii.

In a similar way an increased forward tilt of the pelvis is produced by *minimal* tightness in the hip flexor muscles. Compensation occurs in the lumbar spine, and the lordosis is increased in order to obtain balance.

Prevention and treatment

Correction must be made for the patient in bed, in the wheelchair or standing by:

1. Strengthening the weaker or less used muscle groups.
2. Stretching the muscles tending to shorten.
3. Maintaining a passive stretch in the overcorrected position for the muscles tending to shorten.
4. Re-education of posture.
5. Corrective sleeping postures.
6. Bracing.
7. Archery.

Corrective sleeping postures

Pillows can be used to support the spine in a corrected position at night. For example, a patient with a long C curve to the left should have sufficient pillows under the thorax when lying on his left side to give maximum correction of the deformity.

Bracing

A spinal brace may be necessary to support the child or adolescent with a bad posture in sitting or standing. Occasionally an adult may also need a brace for this purpose.

Archery

Archery is an excellent exercise for the back and shoulder girdle muscles (see Fig. 17.1a). Correction of a scoliosis may be obtained at the full draw position. If the scoliosis is a simple one, the bow is held by the arm on the side of the concavity, as maximum strength is required by the arm pulling the bow string.

If the scoliosis is complex an X-ray is taken at full draw using each arm in turn to see if correction can be obtained.

Surgery

Surgical procedures may be indicated in a few selected cases (Roaf, 1972).

OEDEMA

Feet and legs

Due to the poor vasomotor control and loss of muscle tone in the legs, some patients get oedema of the feet, ankles and lower legs when they first start sitting out of bed. This is, of course, severely aggravated if the patient has had a deep venous thrombosis.

Every effort must be made to correct this condition in the early stages so that it does not become chronic.

To stimulate the vasomotor system, the legs are elevated several times during the day, and if necessary the bed is elevated at night. Besides being elevated in the physiotherapy department the patient should be responsible to put his feet up on a chair at appropriate times during the day, for example, at meal times, in the occupational therapy department and while watching television. The therapist should work out a suitable programme with the patient.

Only if this procedure fails to reduce the swelling after 3–4 weeks are elastic stockings supplied. These are more frequently necessary for patients who have had a deep venous thrombosis. Full length stockings are given. The patient may need to spend 24–48 hours in bed with the foot of the bed elevated to disperse the oedema before measurements for the stockings can be taken.

Hands

Patients with high lesions sometimes develop oedema in the hands. This is again due to impairment of the vasomotor control with consequent loss of vasoconstriction in the blood vessels and poor venous return. This always occurs below the level of the lesion. If the oedema is not dispersed, the collagen deposit is changed into fibrous tissue and contractures develop.

Elevation. To reduce the oedema, the hands are kept in elevation day and night except during occupational therapy and physiotherapy sessions.

Passive movements. Forced passive movements to oedematous joints can only cause trauma and encourage the formation of contractures. Therefore movements are given to affected joints with extreme care and full range is obtained only when the swelling is reduced, which may take half-an-hour or several days. Treatment is given several times a day taking care to maintain full range of all the nonaffected joints. After an initial period of elevation, Boxing Glove splints may be used if desired to keep the swelling down.

In tetraplegic patients usually over the age of 30, oedema followed by contractures of the metacarpophalangeal and interphalangeal joints sometimes occur in spite of regular and intensive treatment. In these cases the joints often resemble rheumatoid arthritic joints. They are red and shiny as well as swollen. The aetiology of this complication is still obscure.

When the disease has ceased to be active, treatment can be given as described for contractures.

OSTEOPOROSIS

Research into the physiology of bone formation and absorption has shown that the mineral metabolism associated with atrophy of the muscular and skeletal systems changes as a result of prolonged bed rest. These changes are emphasised when the bed rest is combined with immobilisation. Considering the inevitable immobility of the paralysed limbs, it is not surprising that osteoporosis is present to some degree, below the level of the lesion, in all tetraplegic and paraplegic patients. The degree of osteoporosis is considerably increased by chronic infection from any cause.

Spontaneous fractures

Osteoporotic bone is rarified bone and therefore easily fractured. Fractures can occur as a result of exceptionally minor injuries and are therefore referred to as 'spontaneous' fractures. For example, a patient who has had his paraplegia for some time may fracture his femur whilst dressing or turning over in bed, or a child may receive a simple knock in school.

The therapist can easily fracture an osteoporotic limb through careless handling when giving strong and extensive passive movements, particularly if contractures are present.

Due to his lack of sensation the patient may be unaware that a fracture has occurred until the area becomes swollen, or until he feels unwell, or has a fever. The therapist and the nursing staff should inspect the legs for any swelling and report abnormal findings to the doctor immediately.

The fractures are generally treated conservatively using well-padded splints. The splint is removed daily and the limb inspected for any areas of excessive pressure or skin damage. Before reapplication of the splint the padding is renewed.

Where possible, passive movements are continued to maintain joint range.

Treatment of osteoporosis

General condition

The patient is turned frequently to aid the circulation and is given a high protein diet with added Vitamin D.

Physiotherapy

When the patient is in bed passive movements are given to the paralysed limbs and resisted exercises to the arms to increase the circulation.

When the patient is up in the wheelchair he is given intensive physiotherapy including long periods of standing and walking.

PAIN

The therapist is not directly involved with the clinical significance of the different types of pain in paraplegia and tetraplegia. There are three types of pain, however, with which she may be concerned and about which she should be informed:

1. pain due to periarticular and muscular contractures
2. nerve root pain
3. referred pain.

Pain due to periarticular and muscular contractures

This pain is always found above the level of the lesion, most frequently in complete lesions of the cervical cord, and is due to faulty positioning and lack of movement. Trauma to the cervical roots may cause some root irritation initially, but continuing pain appears to be due to contractures around the shoulders and shoulder girdle. The treatment given is general mobilisation as for any contracted joint where sensation is unimpaired. It must be borne in mind that the patient's general condition and morale at this time is often poor and his pain tolerence low. Rough handling or indiscriminate stretching of a joint sets up involuntary protective spasm, the patient loses confidence and the desired result is considerably delayed.

Nerve root pain

Patients with conus and cauda equina lesions complain of attacks of pain, often of wavelike intensity, with shooting, stabbing or burning sensations down the legs. There is a high incidence of this pain in incomplete lesions. They often adopt a characteristic attitude during an attack, bowed forward over the knees with one hand gripping the thigh and the other behind the neck. The acute pain usually lasts a few seconds. The number of attacks per day varies considerably from patient to patient and even from day to day in the same patient. The pain is due to post-traumatic changes around the damaged spinal cord and roots. Only mild analgesics are prescribed as drugs are quickly habit-forming in these cases. Intensive physiotherapy is given, including some form of sport. In a number of cases, the condition shows some spontaneous improvement as the patient learns to tolerate his pain by diversional activities. Work is a good antidote. Intractable root pain is occasionally treated by alcohol block with satisfactory results.

Patients with complete lesions of the mid-thoracic and thoraco-lumbar cord sometimes develop a band of hyperpathia around the level of the lesion. The patient complains that there is a tight band around his chest, and occasionally it is so hypersensitive that he cannot bear anything to touch his skin.

Referred pain

Patients with cervical and high thoracic lesions can experience pain in the shoulder region when any abnormal visceral activity occurs. Impulses are carried from the paralysed to the non-paralysed area via the phrenic nerve. For example, a patient with a C_4 lesion had a haematemesis due to a perforated ulcer. On looking back at the therapist's notes it was seen that the patient had complained of nausea and pain across the upper part of the shoulders for at least 2 weeks previously.

Patients with cervical lesions can suddenly develop severe frontal headache. This may be due to overdistension of the bladder and should be investigated without delay.

PARA-ARTICULAR OSSIFICATION

'A special form of para-articular ossification exclusively of non-infectious or traumatic aetiology has been repeatedly observed in both complete and incomplete paraplegics and tetraplegics below the level of the lesion.' (Guttman, 1973.)

There are numerous publications from many parts of the world on this subject, but the aetiology and pathology of the disease remain obscure.

The development of bone in the connective tissue always occurs below the level of the lesion and rarely after the first 6 months post injury. The areas most commonly affected are the hips, knees and elbows and the medial aspect of the femur. The joints themselves are not affected, but the ossification can become massive enough to cause an extra-articular ankylosis.

The degree of ossification which occurs before the disease burns itself out varies considerably. Some patients have very little residual loss of joint range whilst others have severe loss of function and independence.

The therapist is often the first member of the team to notice the onset of the disease. When moving the limb she becomes aware that the joint involved does not feel quite normal. Although there is no real resistance to movement, the joint does not 'feel' clear and free. It is as though the movement were taking place through sponge. At this very early stage there will be no radiological evidence and there may not be any visible evidence, just the awareness of a vague abnormality on moving the limb. Swelling may occur within a few days and possibly some erythema.

Early X-ray evidence shows cloudy patches in the muscles involved but this may not show up for a further 2–3 weeks, and by this time there will be some joint stiffness.

As the disease progresses X-ray shows calcerous desposits in the para-articular tissues and finally dense ossification of the ligaments, fasciae and muscles surrounding the joints.

Current physiotherapy

In the initial stage when the joint feels 'spongy' and the area may be red and swollen, passive movements to that joint are discontinued until the inflammation has subsided. This will take approximately a week; passive movements are then re-commenced. The limb is moved slowly and carefully two or three times only through as full a range as possible. No forced movements are given, but every effort is made to maintain the range.

When the disease becomes less active, after approximately 4-8 weeks, the passive movements and general activity are increased and careful effort is made to increase the joint range.

It is thought that *vigorous* passive movements given to patients with acute lesions may result in small haemorrhages in muscle and connective tissue and that this may be a contributory factor in the formation of para-articular ossification. Therefore, all passive movements must be given carefully especially once this disease has been diagnosed.

Surgery

Gross para-articular ossification interferes with joint range and, as a result, with independence. If severe it may even interfere with a comfortable sitting posture in the wheelchair.

To restore some independence operations have been performed to remove the bone, but surgery is only considered after the disease has completely burnt itself out which is usually 18 months–2 years after onset. Recurrence of ossification is not uncommon even after this time lapse.

PRESSURE SORES

The effects of pressure and its prevention are described in Chapter 6.

The treatment of established pressure sores

Conservative treatment

1. Relieve pressure

The first essential step in treating a pressure sore is to relieve totally and continuously the pressure on the sore. This means complete bed rest for patients who are already ambulant or wheelchair bound.

The patient must be *turned* every 3 hours *day and night* to prevent further sores from developing on unaffected areas, and *positioned* in such a way that no weight is thrown on the sore or sores. Rings around the heels to relieve localised pressure are contra-indicated. The area of skin under the ring may receive sufficient pressure to cut off the blood supply to the area in the centre, which is the area most at risk.

A low air loss bed facilitates positioning a patient with multiple sores, a sorbo pack bed or pillow packs spaced as for sorbo packs can be used on top of an ordinary mattress.

If pressure is not relieved over the sore any other measures taken will prove unsuccessful.

2. General treatment

Blood transfusions may be required to keep the haemoglobin level in the upper limits of normal.

3. Local treatment

All slough and necrotic tissue is radically excised by the doctor in charge of the case. This prevents the toxic effects which result from the absorption of dead tissue into the blood stream. A wide range of lotions is used, including local antibiotics in solution, and the dressing is completely sealed off with wide porous elastoplast.

4. Surgical procedures

Various surgical procedures may be considered in selected cases.

Physiotherapy

Passive movements

Passive movements are given to the paralysed limbs to improve the circulation and to prevent contractures.

Passive movements to the lower limbs are re-commenced after surgery when the surgeon considers it advisable. As a general rule the cases can be divided into those with severe spasticity and those with flaccid lesions.

If the patient has severe spasticity or if any one movement causes violent spasm, all movements are avoided until the scar is healed.

If the lesion is flaccid or the patient has minimum spasticity, it may be possible to commence moving the knees and feet after a week to 10 days.

Initially very gentle movements only are given. Whilst moving the joints involved the therapist watches the scar to avoid excessive tension. The range of any movement which looks potentially danger- ous is increased with *extreme* caution to avoid breakdown of the wound.

Grease massage

The pliability of the skin is an important factor when excision of the sore is considered. The more pliable the surrounding tissues the easier the approximation of the skin following the excision. When necessary daily massage with lanolin is given to a wide area surrounding the sore. Deep finger kneading increases the circulation and improves the elasticity and mobility of the skin and subcutaneous tissues.

In a few selected cases grease massage is given to free adherent scar tissue from underlying structures and so reduce tension and the risk of a breakdown. Extreme care must be taken to avoid damaging the delicate tissue.

Exercise

The patient is encouraged to pull a chest expander or lift weights of suitable strength several times every hour to maintain strength in the arms and upper trunk.

Chest therapy

Pre- and post-operative therapy is given if a general anaesthetic is used for any surgical procedures.

Pressure consciousness

The patient must be educated, or re-educated, in 'pressure consciousness'.

Transfers

In spite of any previous rehabilitation, once the patient is mobile all transfers are checked to see that due care is taken when lifting and moving the limbs.

SPASTICITY

During the period of spinal shock following complete transverse section of the cord, there is flaccid paralysis of all muscles below the level of the lesion. Subsequently the isolated cord resumes some autonomous function and the motor paralysis becomes spastic.

The heightened reflex activity of the isolated cord is demonstrated by increased tone in the muscles, and brisk tendon reflexes. The ensuing degree of spasticity varies. In some cases it may remain mild, in others the afferent stimuli, uninhibited by higher centres, 'spreads out' in the isolated cord and a mass response of muscle action ensues. This can produce any combination of muscle spasm, for example, total flexor or extensor patterns, or alternating flexor and extensor spasticity, or flexion of the knees with extension of the hips.

The increased muscular tension leads to an uneven distribution of pressure on joint cartilage. This may result in destruction of cartilage, capsular contractures or partial dislocations of varying degrees.

Treatment of established spasticity

A combination of the following methods may be used:

physiotherapy
chemotherapy
surgery.

Certain factors stimulate spasticity and these are excluded before deciding on a course of treatment:

1. Distension of internal organs below the level of the lesion, i.e. bladder and bowels.
2. Septic conditions, such as urinary tract infections, or infected pressure sores.
3. Contracted tendons and joints, which reduce the threshold of irritability of the stretch reflex.
4. Local skin lesions, ingrowing toe nails, etc.

When considering treatment the following facts are borne in mind:

1. Fatigue has a depressant effect on spasticity.
2. Muscle accommodates to prolonged stretch.
3. Posture influences reflexes.
4. Spasticity is influenced by emotional factors.

Physiotherapy

Passive movements

These are always given to maintain mobility in all structures.

Prolonged passive stretching

The stretch may be given manually, or by utilising one of the stretch positions as for contractures, or in the standing position.

Hydrotherapy

Passive movements and swimming exercises in a heated pool reduce spasticity in 90% of patients.

Reflex inhibiting postures

These may be useful to reduce spasticity or maintain relaxation during treatment. The position adopted in bed can be used to reduce spasticity. For example, sleeping prone for 3 or 4 hours reduces flexor spasticity in the lower limbs.

Standing and walking

Weight-bearing reduces spasticity. However, in some severely spastic cases the standing position may be impossible without first reducing the spasticity by some other means, e.g. passive movements, a passive stretch, hydrotherapy.

Ice therapy

Immersion in ice is useful for reducing spasticity in the extremities. Ice towels are effective where the spasticity is associated with contracture but have not proved valuable in treating the large muscle groups for spasticity alone.

Chemotherapy

Chemotherapy is used in the following ways:

Drug therapy

Antispasmodic drugs can be used with some effect on certain patients, although their effectiveness in reducing severe spasticity is extremely limited. They are usually prescribed with caution only after a period of physiotherapy has proved insufficient, as the side-effects, notably that of sedation, can affect the patient's rehabilitation.

Local temporary block

Injections of phenol locally into spastic muscles temporarily reduces the spasticity and allows other forms of treatment to be used to good effect. The most common sites are the gastrocnemius, hamstrings, triceps and pectoral muscles.

Intrathecal injection of alcohol

An injection of alcohol into the spinal canal produces a permanent central block of all nervous conduction to and from the cord. It is therefore severely destructive and interferes with vasomotor control and bladder and sexual function. For this reason, it is used rarely and only in cases of intractable spasticity when all other methods have failed and the increased tone is making life intolerable for the patient.

Surgery

Surgical procedures on peripheral structures are preferred to those performed on the cord or roots.

Methods used to reduce spasticity include diminishing the contraction potential of the muscle by elongating the tendon, or by severing the nerve supplying a large muscle group, and occasionally by simple tenotomy.

In certain cases with complete or incomplete lesions it appears that one muscle 'triggers' off the spastic pattern. In these cases a surgical procedure may be performed to block conduction to the 'trigger' muscle. In most cases the result is an overall reduction in spasticity.

The following surgical procedures are frequently performed:

elongation of the Achilles tendon
obturator neurectomy
iliopsoas release by iliopsoas myotomy (Michaelis, 1964)
tenotomy of the hamstrings
tenotomy of the extensor hallusis longus
tenotomy of the toe flexors.

17

Sport

THE THERAPEUTIC VALUE OF SPORT

Clinical sport has an important contribution to make in the rehabilitation of patients with spinal cord injury. It assists in restoring the patient's strength, balance, co-ordination and endurance. It stimulates activity of mind and encourages self-confidence. Some patients were enthusiastic sportsmen before becoming disabled, and once introduced to sport in a wheelchair, will continue when they leave hospital. Sports clubs provide a useful opportunity for mixing with the local community.

Swimming, archery and table tennis are particularly valuable during rehabilitation, but many other sports such as fencing, bowling, field and track events, slalom, dartchery and, in particular, wheelchair basketball have become very popular.

SWIMMING

The pool

To enable patients to swim, the pool must be a reasonable length, possibly a minimum of 8 m. If different depths are required a sloped floor is preferable to steps. Skin damage can easily occur against the hard edges of steps as the paralysed legs trail in the water. As it is generally found that cold water increases spasticity, the water temperature is kept high, that is, between 90° and 96°F or 32° and 36°C. At this temperature spasticity is reduced in the majority of patients.

Hygiene

The pool should have some form of continuous flow system through a filter plant. The chlorine content is maintained and checked twice a day. Samples of the water are cultured regularly. The patient expresses his bladder prior to entering the pool and should have had a satisfactory bowel evacuation.

Entry into the water

Some type of hydraulic lift provides the safest method of entry for all tetraplegic patients and for those patients with lower lesions who are incapable of independent transfer. Active paraplegic patients enter over the side of the pool using a sorbo-rubber pad placed over the edge to protect the skin from the hard surface.

Therapeutic uses

Increase of muscle strength

Swimming increases the strength of all innervated muscles. Motor power in patients with incomplete lesions can be increased by normal hydrotherapy techniques, using water to eliminate gravity or to assist or resist movement.

Improved co-ordination

Co-ordination can be improved by all the strokes used in swimming, in particular by the unilateral strokes.

Reduction of spasticity

This is achieved *passively* through the heated water, passive movements and passive stretching and *actively* through swimming.

Increased respiratory function

Swimming prone increases the activity of the diaphragm and consequently lung volume in patients with cervical cord lesions because of the need to hold the breath in this position.

Reduction of contractures

Passive stretching of contractures is often facilitated by the heated water.

Psychological and social aspect

Mobility in the water is often the only experience of unaided body movement within the environment that most paralysed patients enjoy. Consequently a new enthusiasm is often noted when pool activities are commenced. Swimming fosters the growth of independence and self-expression. It also provides a further opportunity to mix with the able-bodied; many patients enjoying swimming with family and friends.

Swimming instruction

The Halliwick method of teaching independence in the water is largely used in the United Kingdom as a recreational activity, but it has great value also in the therapeutic field (Martin, 1981). The objective of this method is water safety leading to independent freedom of movement in water which is achieved with no help other than a close instructor/swimmer relationship (Martin, 1981). This method suggests that the swimmer should first adjust to the water and then learn to change his position in the water so that he can always move himself into a position in which he is able to breathe.

Rolling

To roll in the water the swimmer turns his head to one side, e.g. the left, and moves one arm, e.g. the right, across his body causing him to tip over until he is face down in the water. The same procedure is repeated to continue the roll to bring the swimmer face upwards again. The 360° roll needs to be practised until it can be done with ease.

Independence in the water is first achieved on the back, the prone position being more difficult to maintain without muscle power at the hip joints. Symmetrical strokes are taught initially, as asymmetrical activity causes the paralysed limbs to roll and the patient finds difficulty in maintaining a straight course.

Instruction for patients with thoracic or lumbar lesions

When supine in the water the paralysed portion of the body lies at an angle of 45° from the site of the fracture. To compensate for the paralysed limbs the head needs to be well extended.

Back stroke

The therapist supports the patient under the neck; the patient, maintaining his head in extension, moves his arms simultaneously away from the sides with the elbows flexed. He then extends the elbows and brings the arms back to *mid-line*, with the thumbs just breaking the surface of the water. Because the hips are lower in the water the body will be pushed upwards if the arms are brought back to the *sides*. Similarly, when the patient relaxes the stroke, his body will sink again. In this way, a vertical as well as a horizontal component to the movement is produced with consequent wasted effort. Once the patient has become accustomed to his position in the water, the 'skulling' stroke is expanded, and the arms are brought out of the water close to the head, as in the Old English back stroke. To prevent his head submerging when the arms are in full elevation, the patient must relax his extended head for a second or two.

Breast stroke

The position of the body when the patient is prone in the water resembles an inverted U, with the head submerged and the buttocks floating to the surface. To counteract this tendency initially the patient is taught to do the breast stroke with his head constantly out of the water, as strong extension of the head and upper trunk is needed to keep the buttocks submerged.

The therapist assists the patient with one hand under his chin and the other pressing down on his buttocks. As the patient becomes aware of his position in the water, the chin support is withdrawn. Later the pressure on the buttocks is gently released and the patient must work hard to maintain the necessary extension. When this is achieved the patient beings to swim with his head under water for several strokes in the usual way. He must, however, *start* to extend his head much sooner than the able-bodied breaststroke swimmer. The head of the paraplegic swimmer will be forced under water just before his hands are level with his shoulders.

Unilateral strokes (crawl)

Without the necessary leg movement to prevent it, the lower half of the body will roll during a unilateral stroke. The roll can be prevented during back crawl by making small paddling movements with the nonstroke arm as the stroke arm pulls down. Compensation cannot be made in this way during front crawl, and few patients do it successfully.

Instruction for patients with cervical lesions

Patients with functional use of latissimus dorsi and triceps swim in the same way as the patients with lower lesions. Patients with lesions at C_6 can occasionally become independent swimmers, but the majority, although capable of swimming alone, need an attendant in case difficulties arise.

Rolling

See page 230.

Back stroke

To gain extension at the elbow without triceps the arm must be kept in lateral rotation and it can be lifted only a few degrees above shoulder level. As the arm returns to the water and pulls down, water pressure will keep the elbow straight.

Swimming prone

Without triceps the true movements of the breast stroke are impossible. The patient with a lesion at C_{5-6} *pulls* his arms through the water towards his body using biceps, deltoid and the clavicular head of pectoralis major. While the patient is swimming face down it is important that the thrapist keeps one hand on the patient's shoulder where he has sensation. Initially, most patients will only be able to swim two or three strokes, but within six or seven sessions this can be increased up to an average of 8–10 m.

Leaving and returning to the side of the pool

To leave the side the patient lies parallel with the side of the pool with the head extended and pushes off gently, with the arm just on the surface of the water. To return to the side the patient swims in parallel with, and as close as possible to, the side of the pool, keeping the near side arm under the surface of the water. He then rapidly flings the arm into the overflow trough and strongly flexes his neck. To maintain this position, paddling movements are performed with the free arm by pulling the water towards the body, as in the breast stroke movement.

Incomplete lesions

Patients with incomplete lesions with weak, scattered muscles and patchy sensation can gain strength and co-ordination from using all the available swimming strokes.

ARCHERY

From both the medical and recreational aspects archery has proved to be an ideal sport for patients with spinal cord injury.

Therapeutic value

Increase of muscle strength

Archery develops and strengthens the essential muscles of the paraplegic patient, that is, erector spinae, deltoid, pectorals, rhomboids, trapezius and latissimus dorsi. (Fig. 17.1a)

Balance, control and co-ordination

When the bow arm is lifted and the centre of gravity consequently altered, skilled balance is required to maintain the erect posture. Initially patients with high thoracic lesions may need to bring the buttocks slightly forward in the chair and lean heavily against the backrest to achieve sufficient stability. As the balance improves the upright posture is resumed.

Accurate marksmanship requires control, dexterity, and judgment and demands fine co-ordination of the eye, hand and arm.

Correction of scoliosis

Archery is used as a corrective exercise for many patients with scoliosis. The string is drawn by the arm on the side of the convexity, irrespective of the dominant eye, to strengthen the weaker muscles. For a simple scoliosis the correction is usually obvious. With a multiple scoliosis, X-rays taken while sitting at rest and again at full draw are essential to confirm that the correct arm is being used to draw the string.

Social value

The disabled and the able-bodied can meet on equal terms. The wheelchair archer can join a club for the able-bodied which provides a further opportunity for integration with the local community.

Archery for patients with cervical cord lesions

Special equipment is necessary to enable the tetraplegic patient to shoot.

The release

To release the arrow without finger flexion or extension a hook device is used. A small hook at the end of a metal splint is strapped to the palmar surface of the middle finger and across the wrist of the drawing hand (Fig. 17.2). To release the string the archer slightly

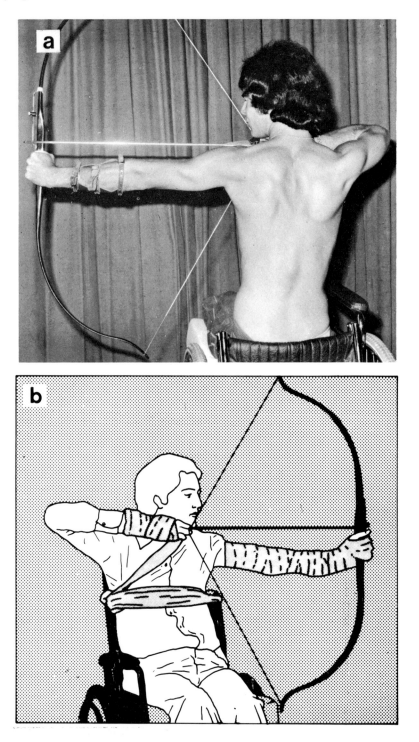

Fig. 17.1   Archery. (a) Patient with a complete lesion below T_{10}. (b) Patient with a complete lesion below C_6.

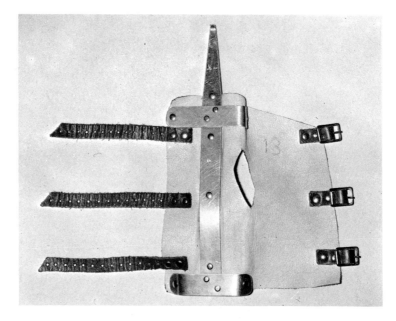

Fig. 17.2 Archery hook.

pronates his forearm. Pronation gives greater accuracy as supination allows gravity to act on the unstable forearm. This causes the elbow to drop and results in inaccurate shooting. With the appropriate training, archers of ability who use the hook release can reach the longest international distance of 90 m.

The bow arm

The patient without triceps needs a splint to maintain the elbow in extension. If the wrist extensors are weak a wrist splint is frequently necessary to prevent the wrist being forced into flexion by the tension of the bow. The bow needs bandaging into the hand. To gain the necessary stability, all patients with cervical cord lesions need to be tied into the chair. The tie is usually placed around the upper thorax and tied to the chair handle on the side of the drawing arm (Fig. 17.1b).

DARTCHERY

This game, played in pairs, was developed for paraplegic patients. Bow and arrows are used to shoot at a target face which is a replica of a dartboard. The target is set at a distance of 15 m from the players and the rules are basically the same as those governing dart play.

TABLE TENNIS

Therapeutic value

1. Improved co-ordination, especially that of eye and hand.
2. Improved agility in the wheelchair.

The loss of sensation and lack of balance make the patient fearful of falling during his early days in a wheelchair. Consequently the patient is often rigid — unwilling to move any part of his body except his head. In his desire to hit the ball this fear is gradually forgotten and the patient comes to realise that he can move about within the chair without either tipping it or falling out. The patient is taught to play with the chair stationary in the centre of the backline. The rules of play are the same as for the able-bodied, with the exception of the 'alternate shot rule' for doubles. This rule is amended so that either partner can return any shot except when receiving service. Patients with cervical cord lesions also enjoy table tennis. Those without finger movement need the bat bandaged, or strapped into the hand. To play backhand shots those without triceps use outward rotation of the shoulder.

SLALOM

Training in wheelchair management is improved by competition over slalom courses. The obstacles will include ramps and turns in narrow confines. Penalties are given for touching, as well as moving, any of the marker bouys.

BASKETBALL

Wheelchair basketball is a fast and exciting game which calls for team work and accurate control of the body, chair and ball. Mobility, strength, endurance and dexterity in wheelchair management are developed. It is a game for those patients with a good functional grip, as accurate and immediate control of the chair is essential. A less active form of this game, volleyball, can be played by patients in their first period of rehabilitation.

FIELD EVENTS

Perfect timing, rhythm and balance are required to achieve a good throw. As extreme mobility of the spine is necessary, this sport may be withheld from patients during their initial period of rehabilitation.

SNOOKER

This game provides excellent co-ordination activity, particularly for patients with cervical cord lesions.

AQUA-LUNG DIVING

Aqua-lung diving is a recent addition to the group of sports open to the person disabled by spinal cord injury. Paralysed sportsmen can dive to moderate depths with aqua-lung apparatus although underwater swimming comes within the definition of 'high risk' or adventure sports even for the able-bodied. If the sport is to be promoted safely close co-operation between those medical practitioners who understand the disability and aqua-lung diving experts is essential. The safety factor is always lower for a disabled sportsman and such a person should dive only when accompanied by two able-bodied experienced divers as companions. This sport is most suitable for those with complete paralysis resulting from trauma. Those with complete lesions above T_5, or with incomplete lesions or those whose paralysis has been caused by a vascular lesion should not participate in this sport.

RULES

All sports are conducted as far as possible under the rules of the game for the able-bodied; for example, archery under the rules of the Grand National Archery Association and swimming under the Amateur Swimming Association's rules. Books of rules are available which cover all sports played by wheelchair competitors.

THE BENEFIT OF COMPETITIVE SPORT

In one sense all sport is competitive. The sportsman always 'competes' with his past performance. He also competes, consciously or unconsciously, with others taking part in the same swimming session or archery class. However, some go on to compete in open competitions and championships. A profitable physical and psychological stimulus is provided by competitive sport. These activities create a sense of comradeship and help to eliminate any self-consciousness suffered by patients in relation to their disability.

Competitive sport is also of great value in integrating disabled people with the able-bodied community. The facilities of some sports centres are now available for both groups.

The majority of sports open to paralysed sportsmen are unsuitable for open competition with the able-bodied, with the exception of archery, green bowling, snooker and table tennis. Basketball, fencing, field events, swimming, track racing and weight lifting are sports which can be competitive only amongst disabled people.

Competitive sport for patients with spinal cord injury is organised on a national and international level through the Stoke Mandeville Games for the Paralysed and Other Disabled.

18
Resettlement

RESETTLEMENT THROUGH THE SOCIAL WORKER

The social component of rehabilitation is complex. The aim is for each patient to lead as normal a life as possible and, whenever feasible, to return home. Between 70 and 80% of patients with spinal cord injury are able to do so. After obtaining relevant information from members of the rehabilitation team and establishing liaison with the social services department, the social worker, the patient and his family plan for the future.

PSYCHOLOGICAL READJUSTMENT

Psychological readjustment is a most important aspect of rehabilitation. Both the patient and his family need support through discussion to make the necessary mental adjustments to the residual disability. They have many anxieties giving rise to fear, frustration, anger and often a sense of isolation. They will have many questions regarding prognosis, home and family life, sex, employment, rehabilitation and practical environmental and financial problems. It is important to gain the confidence of the patient and his family and to encourage questions if the patient is to receive the help he needs (see Ch. 3).

ACCOMMODATION

The two major practical problems in resettlement are obtaining suitable accommodation and employment. Paraplegic patients, except for those handicapped by age or other illness, are usually able to return to live independently in the community. The majority of tetraplegic patients do return to their own homes, although often with maximum support from the social services and the family.

The home may need to be adapted or it may need an extension. However, it may be totally unsuitable and the only solution is to rehouse in a flat or bungalow. Very few houses are suitable without adaptation as most have small bathrooms or passageways with insufficient turning room for the wheelchair.

Adaptations

The need for adaptation varies considerably in relation to the level of the patient's lesion and to his age and sex. Those adaptations most frequently necessary are to the bathroom facilities and, for female paraplegic patients, to the kitchen. Access for the wheelchair to the toilet and bath or shower is necessary for those patients capable of independent transfer. The housewife may also need adaptations to cupboards, cooker and working surfaces in the kitchen so that she can cook without unnecessary danger.

Free access to the house from outside is essential and those able to drive will need a garage wide enough to accommodate the wheelchair beside the car for independent transfer.

Equipment

Some patients will need very little, if any, special equipment in the home, others may need a great deal. A bed, ripple mattress, hoist, and home nursing equipment, as well as a telephone and environmental Possum, or other environmental control system, may all be necessary for a patient with a high cervical lesion.

Hostels and long-term care

For those patients unable to return home, there are a few hostels which accommodate independent paraplegic patients who can obtain open employment in the area. Accommodation for patients with cervical cord lesions may be found in young chronic sick units, Cheshire homes, geriatric units, voluntary institutions and hostels with sheltered workshops.

TRANSPORT

Both paraplegic and tetraplegic patients can have their own cars converted to hand controls. A patient with a lesion as high as C_6 without triceps can drive a car providing it has automatic transmission. A simple system has been developed in France which enables a patient with paralysis of both lower limbs and one upper limb to drive.

Automatic rented cars can be quickly adapted to accommodate a paraplegic driver, which enhances his possibilities of independence when travelling (Dollfus, 1983).

The mechanisms mentioned in Chapter 12 are available to enable the patient *in* the wheelchair to be lifted either into the driver's or the passenger's seat of the car. This is particularly useful for those in electrically powered chairs who are unable to transfer independently but are able to drive.

EDUCATION

Arrangements can be made for the young student to continue his education and even his examinations during his rehabilitation in hospital. Some patients, both paraplegic and tetraplegic, continue their education in colleges of further education, teacher training colleges and universities. Considerable help and understanding are usually given by the authorities, and more facilities are now being provided for the disabled student in many areas.

EMPLOYMENT

Patients with paraplegia

Future employment is discussed with the patient and the disabled resettlement officer as early as possible. The majority of patients are unable to return to their former employment as most are manual workers. Unemployment rates amongst registered disabled persons are higher than in the working population as a whole. Assessment at an industrial rehabilitation unit may be necessary, followed by retraining at a day or residential training establishment for the disabled. Paraplegic patients have been retrained in a variety of occupations, and others, already in professions or business, have returned to all types of work including surgery. Some demonstrate a lack of motivation; for others state benefits are higher than wages.

Patients with tetraplegia

At present open employment is found by only a few patients with tetraplegia because of the amount of care required and the pressure on both the patient and his family. Some patients find employment in sheltered workshops and others work at home.

FINANCE

Financial assistance may be required by the family of the injured wage-earner, who has no financial resources. The social worker is expert in dealing with the complexities of disability allowances, pension plans and other welfare schemes.

AFTERCARE

Medical and social follow up is essential if long-term resettlement is to be satisfactory. Domiciliary visits provide the opportunity for the patient and family to discuss any difficulties with regard to housing, employment and attitude to the disability, which are found after leaving hospital.

Team work between those working with the patient both inside and outside the hospital is required if the patient is to be integrated into the community. This is the keynote of successful rehabilitation.

Appendices

Appendix 1

MAJOR SEGMENTAL INNERVATION OF THE MUSCLES OF THE UPPER LIMB

C2

+C3   Sternomastoid

C3

+C4   Trapezius

+C5   Levator scapulae

C4   Diaphragm

C5   Rhomboids
Deltoid
Teres minor
Supraspinatus
Infraspinatus
Subclavius

+ C6   Biceps

C6   Brachialis
Supinator
Brachioradialis
Subscapularis
Teres major
Coraco-brachialis

+C7   Serratus anterior
Latissimus dorsi
Extensor carpi radialis longus

+C8   Pectoralis major

C7	Pronator teres
	Pectoralis minor
	Extensor digitorum
	Extensor digiti minimi
	Flexor carpi radialis

+C8   Triceps
       Extensor carpi radialis brevis
       Palmaris longus

C8	Extensor carpi ulnaris
	Flexor carpi ulnaris
	Extensor indicis
	Flexor digitorum profundus
	Flexor digitorum sublimis
	Abductor pollicis longus
	Abductor pollicis brevis
	Opponens pollicis
	Flexor pollicis longus
	Extensor pollicis longus
	Extensor pollicis brevis

+T1   Adductor pollicis

T1	Flexor pollicis brevis
	Abductor dijiti minimi
	Flexor digiti minimi
	Opponens digiti minimi
	Lumbricales
	Interossei

Appendix 2

MAJOR SEGMENTAL INNERVATION OF THE MUSCLES OF THE LOWER LIMB

L1	Psoas minor	
	+L2	Psoas major

L2	Iliacus	
	+L3	Sartorius
		+L4 Adductors

L3		
	+L4	Quadriceps

L4	Obturator externus	
	+L5	Tensor fascia lata
		Tibialis posterior
		+S1 Tibialis anterior
		Extensor hallucis
		Extensor digitorum longus
		Peroneus tertius
		Popliteus

L5	Gluteus medius	
	Gluteus minimus	
	+S1	Quadratus femoris
		Semimembranosus
		Semitendinosus
		Biceps femoris
		Peroneus longus
		Peroneus brevis

S1	Obturator internus
	Gastrocnemius
	+S2 Gluteus maximus
S2	Flexor hallucis longus
	Flexor digitorum longus
	Soleus
	+S3 Interossei
S3	Abductor hallucis
	Adductor hallucis
	Lumbricales
	Abductor digiti minimi

Appendix 3

A ROUGH GUIDE TO THE FUNCTIONAL CONTROL OF JOINTS OF UPPER AND LOWER LIMB

	C_5	C_6	C_7	C_8	T_1
Shoulder	Minimal	Partial	COMPLETE		
Elbow	Minimal	Partial	COMPLETE		
Wrist		Minimal	Partial	COMPLETE	
Hand			Minimal	Partial	COMPLETE

	L_2	L_3	L_4	L_5	S_1
Hip	Minimal	Partial	Partial	COMPLETE	
Knee		Minimal	Partial	COMPLETE	
Ankle			Partial	Partial	COMPLETE
Foot			Minimal	Partial	COMPLETE

Appendix 4

FUNCTIONAL INDEPENDENCE

Segmental level	SELF CARE	WHEELCHAIR MANAGEMENT	TRANSFERS	GAIT
C_4	Type, turn pages— Use telephone— with mouth-stick			
C_5	Type Feed	Manipulate brakes Push on the flat		
C_6	Drink Wash, shave, brush hair Dress upper half Sit up/lie down in bed Write	Remove armrests/footplates Push on sloping ground Turn chair	Chair ↔ bed Chair ↔ car ? with sliding board	
C_7	Turn in bed Dress lower half Skin care	Pick up objects from floor Wheel over uneven ground 'Bounce' over small elevations	Chair ↔ toilet Chair ↔ chair ? Chair ↔ bath	Stand in bars
C_8	Bladder and bowel care	Negotiate kerbs	Chair ↔ bath	Swing-to in bars
T_1-T_5		Balance on rear wheels Pull wheelchair into car	Chair ↔ floor	Swing-to in bars
T_6-T_9				Swing-to on crutches Chair ↔ crutches ? Stairs
$T_{10}-L_1$				All three gaits on crutches Stairs Car ↔ crutches Floor ↔ crutches

Appendix 5

SEGMENTAL INNERVATION OF THE SKIN

Upper limb

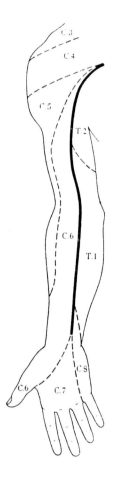

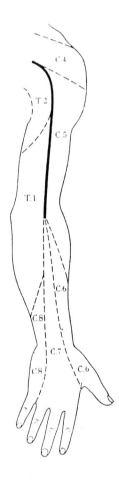

Arrangement of dermatomes on the anterior aspect of the upper limb. The solid black line represents the *ventral axial line*, and the overlap across it is *minimal*. Across the interrupted lines, overlap is considerable.

Arrangement of dermatomes on the posterior aspect of the upper limb. The solid black line represents the *dorsal axial line*, and the overlap across it is *minimal*. Across the interrupted lines, the overlap may be and often is considerable.

Lower limb

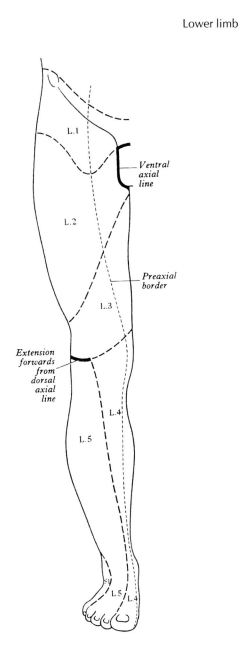

Segmental distribution of nerves of the
lumbar and sacral plexuses to the skin
of the anterior aspect of the lower limb.

Segmental distribution of nerves of the
lumbar and sacral plexuses to the skin
of the posterior aspect of the lower
limb.

Appendix 5 illustrations are reproduced from Gray's Anatomy, 35th edn with permission.

Appendix 6

LIST OF USEFUL ADDRESSES

Association of Carers
Lilac House
Medway Homes
Balfour Road
Rochester
Kent

Association of Crossroads Care
Attendant Schemes Ltd
94 Coton Road
Rugby
Warwickshire
CV21 4LN

The British Sports Association for the Disabled
Stoke Mandeville Sports Stadium for the Paralysed and
    Other Disabled
Harvey Road
Aylesbury
Buckinghamshire

The British Paraplegic Sports Society Ltd
Stoke Mandeville Sports Stadium for the Paralysed and
    Other Disabled
Harvey Road
Aylesbury
Buckinghamshire

Central Council for the Disabled
34 Eccleston Square
London SW1

The Disabled Drivers' Association
4 Laburnum Avenue
Wickford
Essex

Disabled Living Foundation
380–384 Harrow Road
London W9 2HU

Disabled Incomes Group
Queens House
180–182A Tottenham Court Road
London W1P OBD

Joint Committee on Mobility for the Disabled
Wanborough Manor
Wanborough
Guildford
Surrey

National Library of Talking Books for the Handicapped
49 Great Cumberland Place
London W1H 7LH

The Pain Relief Foundation
Walton Hospital
Rice Lane
Liverpool L9 1EA

POSSUM Controls Ltd
11 Fairacres Industrial Estate
Windsor
Berkshire

Spinal Injuries Association
Yeoman House
76 St James Lane
London N10 3DF

Automatic transmissions
Reselco
Invalid Carriages Ltd
262, 264 Kings Street
Hammersmith
London W6

Condom Urinal supplier
GU Manufacturing Co. Ltd
28a Devonshire Street
London W1

Edgerton Stoke Mandeville Tilting and Turning Bed supplier
Edgerton Hospital Equipment Ltd
Tower Hill
Horsham
Sussex

Icarus Easy Transfer Wheelchair Attachment
Icarus Health Aids Ltd
PO Box 324
Industrial Area
Netanya
Israel

Levo Stand-up Wheelchair
Valutec Ltd
Steigstrasse 2
Ch-8610 Uster 3/Zurich

Oswestry Standing Frames
Theo M. Davies
'Argoed'
Glyn Ceiriog
Llangollen
Clwyd. LL20 THN

Sorbo Packs Supplier
Vitafoam Ltd
Don Mill
Middleton
Manchester 4

Stoke Mandeville Urinal supplier
Messrs Down Bros., Mayer and Phelps
Church Path
Mitchum
Surrey

Equipment for the Disabled
Mary Marlborough Lodge
Nuffield Orthopaedic Centre
Oxford OX3 7LD

Yorkhill Chariot
Robert Kellie and Son Ltd
Rutherford Road
Dryburgh Industrial Estate
Dundee DD2 3XF

References and further reading

REFERENCES

Bergstrom E M K, Frankel H L, Galer I A R, Haycock E L, Jones P R M, Rose L S 1985 Physical ability in relation to anthropometric measurements in persons with complete spinal cord lesions below the sixth cervical segment. International Rehabilitation Medicine

Burke D C 1971/72 Spinal cord trauma in children. Paraplegia 9: 1–14

Burke D C 1973/74 Traumatic spinal paralysis in children. Paraplegia 11: 268–276

Cardogo L, Krishnan K R, Polkey C E, Rushton D N, Brindley G S 1984 Urodynamic observations on patients with sacral anterior root stimulators. Paraplegia 22 (4): 201–209

Cheshire D J E 1969/70 The stability of the cervical spine following the conservative treatment of fractures and fracture-dislocations. Paraplegia 7: 193–203

Cheshire D J E, Rowe G 1970/1 The prevention of deformity in the severely paralysed hand. Paraplegia 8: 48–56

Collier P S, Wakeling L M 1982 Diaphragmatic pacing. A new procedure for high spinal cord lesions. Physiotherapy February 68 (2): 47

De Troyer A, Kelly S, Zin Wa 1983 Mechanical action of the intercostal muscles on the ribs. Science 220: 87–88

Frankel H L 1984 Intermittent catheterization. Urologic Clinics of North America 1 (1) February

Dollfus P, Ball J M, Zimmerman M D R, Claudron J 1983 A driving adaptation for tetraplegic persons and a travelling adaptation device for paraplegic persons. Paraplegia 21: 127–130

Duffus A, Wood J 1983 Standing and walking for the paraplegic. Physiotherapy February 79 (2): 45–46

Figoni S F 1984 Cardiovascular and haemodynamic response to tilting and to standing in tetraplegic patients. Paraplegia 22: 99–109

Frankel H L 1967/68 Associated chest injuries. Paraplegia 5: 221–225

Frankel H L 1969/70 Ascending cord lesion in the early stages following spinal injury. Paraplegia 7: 111–118

Frankel H L, Hancock D O, Hyslop G, Melzak J, Michaelis L S, Vernon J D S, Walsh J J 1969/70 The value of postural reduction in the initial management of closed injuries of the spine with paraplegia and tetraplegia. Paraplegia 7: 179–192

Gutmann Sir L, Silver J R 1965 Electromyographic studies on reflex activity of the intercostal and abdominal muscles in the cervical cord lesion. Paraplegia 3: 1–22

Haln H R 1970 Lower extremity bracing in paraplegia with usage follow up. Paraplegia 8 (3): 147–153

Harris P 1967/68 Associated injuries in traumatic paraplegia and tetraplegia. Paraplegia 5: 215–220

Houston J M 1984 Comprehensive education for those concerned with spinal cord injury patients. Paraplegia 22 (4): 244–248

Hughes J T 1984 Regeneration in the human spinal cord: a review of the response to injury of the various constituents of the human spinal cord. Paraplegia 22: 131–137

Maling R G, Clarkson D C 1963 Electronic controls for the tetraplegic (POSSUM) (Patient Operated Selector Mechanism). Paraplegia 1: 161–174

Martin J 1981 The Halliwick method. Physiotherapy October 67 (10): 288–291

McGarry J, Woolsey R, Thompson C W 1982 Autonomic hyperreflexia following passive stretching to the hip joint. Physical Therapy 62 (1) January

Michaelis L S 1964 Myotomy of ilopsoas and obliquus externus abdominis for severe spastic flexion contracture at the hip. Paraplegia 2: 287–294

Mickelberg R, Reed S 1981 Spinal cord lesions and lower extremity bracing on overview and follow-up study. Paraplegia 19: 379–385

Morgan M D L, De Troyer A 1984 The individuality of chest wall motion in tetraplegia. Clinical Respiratory Physiology

Morgan M D L, Silver J R, Williams S J 1984 The respiratory system of the spinal cord patient. Clinical Respiratory Physiology

Pachalski A, Pachalski M M 1984 Programme of active education in the psycho-social integration of paraplegics. Paraplegia 22 (4) 238–243

Ray C 1984 Social, sexual and personal implications of paraplegia. Paraplegia 22: 75–86

Ray C, West J 1984 Coping with spinal cord injury. Paraplegia 22: 248–259

Roaf R 1971/72 The significance of horizontal forces in the development and control of spinal deformities. Paraplegia 9: 183–190

Scott B A 1980 The engineering principle and fabrication technique for the Scott-Craig long leg brace for paraplegics. Review of Orthotics and Prosthetics 281–285

Silver J R 1974/75 The prophylactic use of anticoagulant therapy in the prevention of pulmonary emboli in one-hundred consecutive spinal injury patients. Paraplegia 12: 188–196

Silver J R, Moulton A 1969/70 The physiological and pathological sequelae of paralysis of the intercostal and abdominal muscles in tetraplegic patients. Paraplegia 7: 131–141

Twatsubo E, Komine S, Yamashita H, Imamura A, Akatsu T 1984 Over-distension therapy of the bladder in paraplegic patients using self catheterization: A preliminary study. Paraplegia 22 (4): 210–215

Walsh J J 1968/69 Intermittent catherization in paraplegia. Paraplegia 6: 168–171

Wing P C, Tedwell S J 1983 The weight bearing shoulder. Paraplegia 21: 107–113

Wyndaele M D 1984 A critical review of urodynamic investigations in spinal cord injury patients. Paraplegia 22: 138–144

FURTHER READING

Bedbrook Sir George (ed) 1981 The care and management of spinal cord injuries. Springer-Verlag, Heidelberg.

Bobath B 1978 Adult hemiplegia, 2nd edn. Heinemann, London

Brain Lord 1969 Clinical neurology, 3rd edn (revised by Roger Bannister) Oxford University Press, Oxford

Burke D, Murray D 1975 Handbook of spinal cord medicine. MacMillan, London

Capildeo R, Maxwell A (eds) 1984 Progress in rehabilitation: paraplegia. MacMillan, London

Cash J 1977 Neurology for physiotherapists, 2nd edn. Faber & Faber, London

Chantraine A, Crieleard J M, Onkelink A, Pirnay F 1984 Energy expenditure of ambulation in paraplegics: Effects of long-term use of bracing. Paraplegia 22: 173–181

Conesa S H 1976 Visual aid to the examination of nerve roots. Bailliere Tindall, London

Conti V R, Calverly J, Shaked W L, Estes M, Williams E H 1982 Anterior spinal artery syndrome with chronic traumatic aortic aneurysm. Annals of Thoracic Surgery 33 (1): 81–85

Fallon B 1979 Able to work. Spinal Injuries Association, London

Fallon B 1982 The sexual lives of disabled people. West Sussex Disabilities Study Unit, Arundel

Foo D, Rossier A B 1983 Anterior spinal artery syndrome and its natural history. Paraplegia 21 (1): 1–10

Foo D, Bigname A, Rossier A B 1982 Post traumatic anterior spinal cord syndrome: pathological studies of two patients. Surgical Neurology 17 (5): 370–375

Gatz A J 1970 Manter's essentials of clinical neuro-anatomy and neurophysiology. Davis, Philadelphia

Glenn W W L 1978 Diaphargm pacing — present status. Pace 1: 357–370

Guttmann Sir L 1973 Spinal cord injuries: comprehensive management and research. Blackwell, London

Guttmann Sir L 1976 Textbook of sport for the disabled. H.M. & M. Publishers, Aylesbury, Bucks

Hale G (ed) 1979 Source book for the disabled. Paddington Press, London

Jay P 1983 Choosing the best wheelchair cushion. Royal Association for Disability and Rehabilitation

Levitt S 1977 Treatment of cerebral palsy and motor delay. Blackwell, London

Malick M H, Meyer C M H 1979 Manual on management of the quadriplegic upper extremity.

Mandelstam D 1977 Incontinence. Heinemann, London

Maxted M J, Dowd G S 1982 Acute central cord syndrome without bony injury. Injury 14 (1): 103–106

Moberg E 1978 The upper limb in tetraplegia: a new approach to surgical rehabilitation. Thieme Stuttgart

Morgan M D L, Gourlay A R, Silver J R, Williams S J, Denison D M 1984 The partitioning of ventilation in tetraplegia by optical mapping. Submitted to thorax

Morgan M D L, Gourlay A R, Silver J R, Williams S J, Denison D M 1984 The contribution of the ribcage to breathing in tetraplegia. Submitted to Thorax

Morse S D 1982 Acute central cervical spinal cord syndrome. Annals of Emergency Medicine 11 (8): 436–439

Norris W, Campbell D 1974 Anaesthetics, resuscitation and intensive care. Churchill Livingstone, Edinburgh

Pratt R 1971 Nursing care of the paraplegic patient. Nursing Times Publications, London

Rasch P J, Burke R K 1971 Kinesaelogy and applied anatomy. Lee & Febiger, Philadelphia

Rogers M A 1978 Paraplegia: A handbook of practical care and advice. Faber & Faber, London

Sha' Keed A (ed) 1981 Human sexuality and rehabilitation medicine: Sexual functioning following spinal cord injury. Williams & Wilkins, Baltimore

Scher A T 1983 Hyper-extension trauma in the elderly: an easily overlooked spinal injury. J. Trauma 23 (12): 1066–1068

Spinal Injuries Association 1980 Nursing management in the general hospital: the first 48 hours following injury. SIA,

Szymanski D, Collier R, Orr S 1983 Central cord syndrome (Clinical conference). Annals of Emergency Medicine 12 (1) January: 45–47

Spinal Injuries Association 1984 Spinal cord injuries: Guidance for general practitioners and district nurses. SIA,

Ungar G H 1971 The care of the skin in paraplegia. The Pracitioner 206: 507–512

Walsh J J 1959 Understanding paraplegia. Tavistock, London

Wilshire E R 1982 Wheelchairs — equipment for the disabled. Oxfordshire Health Authority, Nuffield Orthopaedic Centre, Oxford

Index